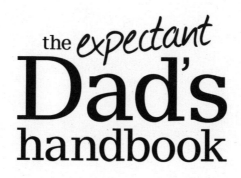

the *expectant*
Dad's
handbook

the *expectant* Dad's handbook

All you need to know about pregnancy, birth and beyond

Dean BEAUMONT

Vermilion
LONDON

7 9 10 8

Published in 2013 by Vermilion, an imprint of Ebury Publishing
Ebury Publishing is a Random House Group company

The Random House Group Limited Reg. No. 954009
Addresses for companies within the Random House Group can be found at
www.randomhouse.co.uk

A CIP catalogue record for this book is available from the British Library

The Random House Group Limited supports The Forest Stewardship
Council® (FSC®), the leading international forest-certification organisation.
Our books carrying the FSC label are printed on FSC®-certified paper.
FSC is the only forest-certification scheme supported by the leading
environmental organisations, including Greenpeace. Our
paper procurement policy can be found at
www.randomhouse.co.uk/environment

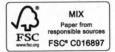

MIX
Paper from
responsible sources
FSC® C016897

Printed and bound in Great Britain by Clays Ltd, St Ives plc

ISBN 9780091948047

Copies are available at special rates for bulk orders. Contact the sales development
team on 020 7840 8487 for more information.

To buy books by your favourite authors and register for offers,
visit www.randomhouse.co.uk

The information in this book has been compiled by way of general guidance in
relation to the specific subjects addressed, but is not a substitute and not to be relied
on for medical, healthcare, pharmaceutical or other professional advice on specific
circumstances and in specific locations. Please consult your GP before changing,
stopping or starting any medical treatment. So far as the author is aware the
information given is correct and up to date as at January 2013. Practice, laws and
regulations all change, and the reader should obtain up to date professional advice on
any such issues. The author and publishers disclaim, as far as the law allows, any
liability arising directly or indirectly from the use, or misuse, of the information
contained in this book.

To Oren, my little boy, whose birth started the journey; to Willow, whose birth reinforced so many of my beliefs; and to my, at this point, unborn child, who will cause Daddy to practise what he preaches.

Most importantly, to my beautiful wife and a wonderful mum, Steph – without her support, patience, ideas, know ledge, editorial skills and the mum's perspective, neither DaddyNatal nor this book would exist.

Contents

Congratulations – You're a Dad!

Yes, it's true: whether you have just found out you're having a child, or you are further down the road and are already a dad, there is so much you can get involved in – now! This book is all about the pregnancy, birth and those all-important first couple of weeks after your baby is born – from the dad's point of view.

I'm Dean Beaumont, the first professional male antenatal educator in the UK and founder of DaddyNatal, a company that runs antenatal classes just for dads. I have two children: my son, Oren, and my daughter, Willow, and over the years I have worked with thousands of families in preparation for parenthood.

I am absolutely passionate about supporting dads to become better prepared for fatherhood. From us dads learning how we impact on the development of our baby before he has even been born to understanding some of our innate instincts, such as our 'fix-it reflex' (see page 78), which can be detrimental when supporting our partner through labour, we men deserve to have access to the information that will enable us to become more positively involved in the pregnancy, birth and early days as a parent. One of the key features of my work with men is defining our roles – I call this being 'protector' and 'advocate' for our partner/baby/family, and giving us the tools and understanding of the context to be able to see this through, in a way that doesn't just make sense to us blokes, but isn't deadly boring either!

Becoming an antenatal teacher was not a path I ever envisaged taking. Before the arrival of my first child, I was working in the building industry and would probably have said my passion was motorbikes! Back then birth and babies were not things that were on my radar. However, the birth of my son, Oren, was pretty life-changing. I thought I was well informed as an expectant father; I'd been to antenatal classes with my other half and had read a couple of books (after being nagged about being more involved!). However, when the big event came it was not as straightforward as I had imagined. I realised I didn't know what to do to help things along and to help my partner cope, or how to advocate for her when it became necessary. This, in itself, was a shock, as I am a pretty confident sort of guy. However, in the environment of the labour and birth I was totally out of my comfort zone. This led to memories of the birth of my son being tainted with feelings of guilt for not being better prepared.

Within a few months of our son's arrival, we found we were pregnant again. This gave me the opportunity to revisit the classes and books I had used to prepare for the birth of my son, and to work out what it was I had missed the first time around. And that's when I realised it – all these resources were, in fact, letting dads down. The antenatal classes were very mum-orientated, with little tailored advice for the dads. The books were either, again, quite woman-orientated or if they were aimed at dads they were quite gimmicky, with an overly 'humorous' or light writing style, at the expense of proper, useful information.

Given that numerous studies show that birth partners (whether the dad, a relative or a doula) have a huge impact on labour and birth and that fathers are so important to child development, I thought it was bonkers that there were no good resources specifically for men to fulfil their role as birth partners. So I set off to train to become an antenatal educator, to help other men to be better informed when their time came to being fathers and to help them to become fully hands-on in helping their partners. DaddyNatal was created. We started off with the first few classes being held in fantastic pubs, who loaned me rooms for free, and we would get a few guys turning up. Our approach was no-nonsense, practical and informative, providing the essential information for dads in a way that was relevant and made sense. Dads loved the style of the class and our reputation quickly started to develop; in 2011 we were awarded a contract to run the classes with Peterborough City Hospital. We still run classes for them today and have had hundreds of dads come through our classes in Peterborough alone. Some of their stories and experiences are included in this book, to show you how much of a difference these techniques make to help dads become more confident and involved in birth.

We now have classes running all around the UK, as more and more dads have joined our team as teachers. However, not all dads can access our classes and many more wanted a one-stop resource comprising all the information in our courses, which is why this book has come into being. I decided to write the book that I felt was still missing, so this book aims to cover all the things you dads need to know to help prepare you for pregnancy, birth and fatherhood.

So why should *you* read this book?

This book is for all expectant dads, whether this is your first baby or your fifth. Trust me, even if it is your fifth, there will still be things in here that you didn't know. As Laurie, one of our DaddyNatal teachers, who has five children (he even 'caught', or brought one of them into the world, at an unexpected home birth) said:

'Being present at all five labours and births, I felt that I had been the best birthing partner I possibly could be ... until I learnt the DaddyNatal way. My eyes were opened to all that a father can be and really should be – an informed and supportive birthing partner for his wife or partner. These techniques give fathers the knowledge to support and advocate for their partners, to make the whole birthing experience as calm and empowering as they can.'
– **Laurie, dad of five**

case study

Single dads – you are important too!

This book is written from the perspective of the mum and dad being together – however, this is simply because of the necessity of writing from a single perspective. This does not mean that the information will not be of use to dads who are no longer in a relationship with the mother of their child. All the tips, advice and warnings are relevant and applicable – even if you are no longer together as a couple. You will still effectively both be parenting your baby as a team. While your relationship will have different dynamics and considerations if you are not living together under one roof, it will still experience both the joys and strains of becoming new parents.

I will talk later about the benefits that supportive dads and partners can bring to the development and raising of our children. Remember that your involvement is crucial; whether you are separated from your partner or not, you will have a marked impact on his development.

From an antenatal perspective, you still need to consider all the topics covered in the book. If you are going to be present at the birth, it would be helpful to have discussed birth preferences, so that you can help and support Mum. If you are not going to be present at the birth because Mum does not feel comfortable with you there (although I realise this may be difficult for you), perhaps the book will help to reassure you that there is plenty you can be getting involved with. At the end of the day, birth outcomes have an impact on baby development, so for your baby's sake you want to support Mum. If it will help her to have the best possible pregnancy and birth she can, with the least amount of stress, then not being there is the selfless thing to do for the sake of your child.

If you are not together as a couple now, you may find that some of the ways I have suggested bonding with your baby (see chapter 2) may not be available to you, but there are still plenty that are – so focus on those to establish your own bond instead.

Once your baby has arrived, it is important that you agree an overall parenting strategy with your partner. Make sure you are both clear on the choices you have made for your baby. You need to support each other as you both embark on your parenting journey. You will have individual challenges to face – just as every dad has his own unique challenges in the situation in which he now finds himself – but the overall points discussed throughout the book are still just as relevant to you.

How to use this book

Dads, to make this book easy for you to use, I have divided it into three main sections – pregnancy, labour and birth, and life with your newborn. This is to make it convenient for you to dip in and out of, as and when you need or want to. I suggest reading as much of the book as you can before the birth (you don't want to be reading about how you should already have prepared for your role in labour while you are right in the thick of it!). This will mean that you are confident and prepared for your specific role as Dad and, possibly, as a birth partner.

The Expectant Dad's Handbook will provide you with non-biased and impartial choices, tools and information at every stage. Taking your time to work through the book will help you to get to grips with what is going on and what to expect, give you a clear sense of what your role is and how to confidently fulfil it, for the benefit of everyone involved.

Overall, whatever your situation as a dad, I'm delighted that by picking up this book you are clearly signalling that you want your influence on your child's life to be a positive one – and that's probably the biggest parenting decision you need to make.

Good luck on your journey into fatherhood!

N.B. *Because babies come as boys or girls, to make everything fair I have alternated the use of 'he' and 'she' chapter by chapter, starting with 'he' in the Introduction and Chapter 1.*

A message for mums

Mums, please feel free to read this book too! Although it is obviously aimed at dads, there is a lot of information that you may also find helpful to read. One of the aims of the book is to support your partner to understand a little more about what you will be experiencing and thinking at the different stages of pregnancy, birth and beyond, and how he can best support you.

This is the book both myself and my wife, Steph, wished we had around the times of the births of our own children. We never seemed to understand the other person's position and we started to recognise a pattern of disagreements between us that were shared by other pregnant couples we knew at the time too! From parenting styles to sex, there are common topics where misunderstandings can take place. This book touches on some of these and will give you a heads-up on how both men and women may approach issues differently, and why, which should help to increase understanding and help avoid some of those conflicts in the future!

Steph is an antenatal educator herself and has had a massive input into the DaddyNatal programme and this book, making sure that we get it right in helping dads to understand what their partners are feeling and experiencing. This truly is a book that aims to increase understanding between mums and dads. For you mums, this book will also give you an insight into the thoughts of dads, our natural instincts and our potential impact on pregnancy, the birth and the wellbeing of the baby.

As I am sure you are already well aware, men approach things differently to the way women do. Humour is a bit of a defence mechanism for us and we use it when we are feeling anxious or uncomfortable, to make light of a situation. This is why us blokes can often be found cracking jokes when it comes to discussions to do with labour and birth. Making men aware of this impulse is the first step to dealing with it, so hopefully there won't be any of those 'bad dad joke' moments during your birth – like those you may have seen on TV or heard from friends!

However, it is not all one-way, and something I hope that this book might also show is why mums make statements such as 'You will be at the birth so you can see what I have to go through to have our baby' or 'I want you to see the pain I suffer giving birth'. These are unhelpful to both your partner and yourself. (This may seem shocking, but these are actually real statements that we have heard many mums make over our years of working with parents.) These kinds of comments often come from a very emotional place, but it is important to realise that they only serve to make it difficult to achieve the birth you want to have. Birth partners have been proved to have a massive impact on labour and birth outcomes, and confident birth partners are much more likely to be able to support mums to experience a positive labour and birth. This means that if Dad is going to be your sole birth partner he needs to be prepared for his role and not feel afraid. By reading this book or attending one of our classes (or even better, both) he will be preparing, so just encourage him as he is learning and make sure he knows how much you want him to be there.

When it comes to babies, a lot of us dads want to be hands-on and involved, but we can feel a bit clumsy and sometimes stereotyped as 'not keen to be hands-on'. If we feel as though we are doing it 'wrong' or are being criticised or excluded, then (often subconsciously) we can end up 'opting out' and doing less and less. The number of times parents have reported back to us that they recognise themselves doing this, once they have been made aware of it, is amazing. Having your first baby is a learning process and as two individual parents you are going to do things differently anyway. You are both going to make mistakes – it is part of a natural learning curve. Dads will go through it as well as mums and it's how we eventually become confident about looking after our children.

I remember once my wife, Steph, berating me because I changed a nappy in a sleep-deprived state and I left our son's bits hanging out, which meant that within half an hour his clothes were soaked – he had weed all over himself! Looking back now, it is just an amusing memory, and these little things do happen. They are not the end of the world, and sometimes it's the silly things we do that give us the things to laugh at when we look back over the years of our children's babyhoods.

So please make sure that you give Dad space to look after his baby. Let him do it his own way – let him get it wrong! If he is relying on you for help too much, why not go and have a nice relaxing bath or go out for a walk, so that you give him space? He is a grown-up and he will be able to do it. For some of us new dads our confidence levels are low and we just need a push in the right direction!

In fact, the more time us dads get to spend with our babies, the better. Our partners are often the main focal point of our lives until a baby comes along. Dads and their children can, and do, have wonderful relationships, but there is something very special about that mum-and-baby bond. Us dads are only human and sometimes we get a bit jealous of that amazing connection, feeling a bit left out. Maybe this sounds a little daft, but it is very true. The deeper our connection and involvement with our baby, the less likely we are to feel that way – and the less likely we are to have all the associated disagreements with Mum that come with it!

Ultimately, becoming parents is easier and more fulfilling if you approach it as a team. It is about learning to look out for each other and accepting that you both have different roles to play, which when you put them together creates a fantastic parenting partnership.

For anyone working with expectant parents

I'm delighted that you have decided to pick up this book, as I am passionate about us professionals all continuing to strive to improve our services – to make them more inclusive, relevant and accessible to dads. Dads have such an important role to play in pregnancy, labour, birth and the upbringing of their baby, and they deserve better than to be expected to learn in environments such as antenatal classes and postnatal groups that have historically been targeted at just women. Together we can help to prepare dads for their roles and, in turn, improve the experience and outcomes for many expectant parents.

There are still far too many stereotypes at play around dads being 'useless', with pregnancy being 'nothing to do with them' or them being a 'spare part'. Recent press that has dismissed dads as not deserving to have an opinion on anything related to birth is sad and only demonstrates a total ignorance about the potential of the role of the father and his importance in the family unit. However, together we can start to challenge these stereotypes and misconceptions and break them down.

Although this book is written mainly for dads, it will still be relevant to all birth partners, whether they are a family friend, same-sex partner, relative or doula. Whoever you are, if you are planning to support someone through a birth, make sure that you understand the impact you could have on that birth – because *just being there is not enough*. If you are suffering trauma from your own birth experience or have a very strong view of how birth 'should' be, then those are issues you need to come to terms with first in order to be a positive birth partner.

Michel Odent, the French medical doctor who became well known in the natural childbirth movement as a proponent of water birth, was famously quoted as saying that dads shouldn't be present at the birth of their child. The truth is that men who are not properly prepared can cause problems in the delivery room. *However, it does not have to be this way.* As professionals working with expectant parents, we all have a responsibility to make sure that the father is as prepared as he can possibly be. We should be supporting dads on their own terms, in ways that make sense to *them*. What they do with this support is then up to them, but we should not be letting them down by dismissing them and their potential before the labour has even begun. In addition, if the learning that is provided is not relevant or accessible to dads, then this is not appropriate either and it is also letting them down.

The book will give you some ideas about introducing specific roles to dads and explain a little about the male psyche. Please consider what is outlined here and try to build some, or all, of the approaches into your work with dads; it will be beneficial for everyone involved.

We constantly offer opportunities to join our DaddyNatal team of teachers, as well as study days for professionals working with expectant and new dads. Please visit www.daddynatal. co.uk for information on all the professional training and support that we offer, or get in touch with me directly.

My vision is that one day all dads will have access to support that is tailored to them. Evidence (see the list of studies on page 228) shows us what a critical difference fathers make at the births of their babies and to the lives of their children afterwards. It is time to stop simply *telling* them to be involved, and to start *showing* them positive ways to do it.

section one

Pregnancy

CHAPTER 1

Your pregnancy roadmap

So you and your partner are expecting a baby and you want to be an involved dad! First up, let's give you an idea of what to expect over the nine months of pregnancy.

Pregnancy is one of those points in our lives where our conversations may suddenly become full of pregnancy- and baby-related jargon – from knowing comments such as 'Ah, she's in her first/second trimester' through to questions such as 'Will you be going to the dating scan?', 'Is she having Braxton Hicks?' and 'What position is the baby in?' This chapter will help you understand all of these aspects – and much more!

It's common for dads to feel that during the pregnancy, and even during the birth, there isn't a great deal they can do – however, this is just not true: your role starts now! It's good to know as much as possible about what's going on with your baby's development. So what is a normal pregnancy like and what is happening during the different trimesters? Also what can you do to help with the changes taking place in your partner?

The three trimesters of pregnancy

'Trimesters' are simply the way of referring to the stages of pregnancy and the developments taking place within the various time frames. Pregnancy is divided into three trimesters:

The trimesters of pregnancy

First trimester: 0–12 weeks (months 1–3)
Second trimester: 13–27 weeks (months 4–6)
Third trimester: 28 weeks–birth (months 7–9)

The journey starts here – the first trimester

Baby

For the first few weeks after conception you were probably totally unaware that you had become a dad, but Baby's development was already moving on at a pace. Once the egg is fertilised the baby starts to grow and by around the sixth week it is already around 6 mm (¼ in) long. The most important organs, such as the heart and brain, are already starting to form.

For the rest of the first trimester Baby continues to develop and by the end of the 12 weeks all the major organs will have been formed. Baby will also have started to move – not that your partner is likely to have felt it yet, as Baby is still only about the size of a small plum.

Mum

Early on during the first trimester you will not know that your partner is pregnant (or you may not know until much later on – if it is a surprise!), but you may start to see signs that make you wonder. These could include morning sickness, cravings or your partner suddenly going off her favourite food. She may also suddenly find herself very tired.

Emotionally Mum and Dad tend to be quite different from each other during the first trimester. Mum is likely to be excited, distracted and filled with apprehension at times. She will likely worry about Baby's health and the possibility of miscarriage. Just telling her 'not to worry' is really not going to help: reassure her and be supportive through the first trimester. Don't try to 'solve' or 'fix' the problem (this is a classic male reflex, which I'll be discussing later in Chapter 7); just be there to listen to her and tell her you understand. With the hormone changes taking place in her body, Mum is likely to be going through mood swings, which can be as unnerving for her as for you!

Dad

In all honesty, you will probably feel a brief feeling of excitement, but that's about it for a while. Early pregnancy tends to be a little unreal for us dads at this stage and you may even find yourself completely forgetting about the pregnancy some days; this is all quite normal.

With regards to her pregnancy cravings, you need to do one of two things. If the cravings are for something that won't do her any harm, then get her what she wants – do that midnight run to the supermarket. The chances are that just as you manage to stock up on the one random item she is craving, she will go off it and you will end up with a cupboardful going to waste – I still remember that well! But enjoy the unexpectedness of the pregnancy cravings and the running around to fulfil them, as they are all part of the fun of the pregnancy, and they will be over soon enough. However, if the craving is for something that she really *shouldn't* be having (see the box overleaf), your job is to try to distract her (if that's possible since cravings can be all-consuming!) and find her something else to do or find a substitute.

What foods aren't recommended in pregnancy?

For dads who are cooking some or all of the meals at home, here is the quick low-down on what foods pregnant women should avoid.

Avoid altogether:
- Alcohol
- Any cheeses that are not pasteurised, blue-veined cheese (such as Danish blue, Gorgonzola and Roquefort) and mould-ripened (such as Brie and Camembert)
- Pâté
- Undercooked eggs (white and yolk should be hard)
- Undercooked meat
- Raw shellfish
- Liver

Cut down on:
- Caffeine
- Certain fish, including tuna and oily fish

Don't forget:
- Make sure all fruits, salads and vegetables are washed thoroughly

Milestone

Usually your first scan is at about 12 weeks. This scan checks that everything is okay with your baby and will give you an estimated due date (EDD). Scans are important bonding opportunities and it is pretty amazing to see how your baby is developing, so try to make sure you attend. This could be the moment when you really *do* realise that you are going to have a baby.

When should you tell the world you're pregnant?

You can tell people whenever you feel ready! Many parents choose to wait until the 12-week scan, when they have actually seen their baby on the screen and the risk of miscarriage has dramatically decreased. However, it is a choice that you and Mum need to make together – whether you wish to tell people earlier or wait a little longer. That is your decision!

Picking up pace – the second trimester

Baby

Baby's development is really moving along now. By the end of the second trimester your baby will be approximately 24 cm (9 ½ in) long and weigh in at around 1 kg (2 lb) (equivalent to a bag of sugar!). All of your baby's organs are developed and growing. Around the 16-week mark Baby may start to hear sounds and at around 24 weeks Baby's real hair may start to grow. Week 20 is when it should be possible to tell the gender of your baby by scan – if this is something you want to know. At around week 24 Baby can differentiate sounds and can start to recognise your voice. This is also a time when you may be able to start feeling Baby move if Mum is resting, so try it. Babies tend to be more active when Mum rests too, since when she is moving around all that movement calms them and rocks them to sleep! So bear this in mind and aim to try to feel movements when you can perhaps both sit down together at the end of the day. By the end of the second trimester your baby's fingernails will have formed and he will also have his fingerprints.

Mum

During the second trimester, physical changes to Mum are likely to start to become noticeable as the bump really starts to grow. Hopefully her morning sickness will pass and her appetite will increase, although be aware that for some mums it may not. Mum may also be able to feel slight movements from Baby from as early as the start of the second trimester, although this varies a lot from person to person.

Around the middle of the second trimester Mum may start to experience tightening sensations around the bump – these are, again, normal and are called 'Braxton Hicks' contractions. These are a warm-up for labour; the body is getting the uterine muscle ready and practising contracting. During these Braxton Hicks the cervix does not start to dilate, which is why it is also sometimes referred to as 'false' labour.

Towards the end of the second trimester is when Mum is likely to experience the greatest weight gain. Swelling of her feet and hands is not unusual during this time as is a stuffy nose (and some snoring during sleep!). Again, a round of cravings may ensue towards the end of the second trimester, so get ready for those late-night visits to the supermarket.

Emotionally, Mum will worry less about things going wrong with the pregnancy, but that doesn't mean she will stop worrying altogether! She may start to worry about a range of issues such as the changes to her body, have concerns about being a good mother, whether she'll be able to breastfeed and whether she will cope with labour and birth. With all the changes taking place, Mum will want reassurance from you that she is still loved and that you are there for her and the baby. Again, do not make light of this – you need to be at your reassuring best. The good news is that as the hormones are settling down, her moodiness and irritability should start to subside.

Dad

Your support during the second trimester is important. As your partner's body shape starts to change, she may become self-conscious. It is not a good idea to make jokes about her shape – under any circumstances! If she experiences swelling of her hands and/or feet, try to make it as easy as possible for her to spend time with her feet up. Towards the end of the second trimester is the perfect time to really start to bond and build your relationship with your baby – see chapter 2 for more on this. The benefits of doing this for all three of you are great, so it's well worth putting in the effort.

Your emotions tend to start to catch up with your partner's at this point. You are likely to feel excited, distracted and even begin to have concerns of your own. You may now start to worry about both the health of your baby and partner as you become aware of the physical changes taking place. You may also worry about the changes to the family unit once Baby joins you and the fear of feeling jealous or of being 'left out'. All of these feelings are totally normal, but you need to deal with these concerns rather than just ignore them. More is explained in chapter 3 on men's fears.

Milestone

You and your partner will have the opportunity to go for a second scan at around 20 weeks. The primary focus of this scan is to check Baby's anatomy and make sure he is developing normally. Again, this is a really good opportunity to bond with your baby, and if you have attended the first scan already you will be amazed at how much he has developed since then. Make sure you ask for a couple of scan pictures to take home with you!

The third trimester

Baby

Your baby is really starting to gain weight now and is beginning to look a lot more like a newborn! He will be opening and closing his eyes and also possibly starting to suck his thumb. All of his organs are continuing to mature and his lungs are starting to fully develop.

As Baby grows he is starting to run short of space in the womb, so his movements feel different to you if you lay your hand on your partner's tum. However, it is very important that you both keep monitoring Baby's movements, and if you think that they are slowing down, that you talk to your midwife. Reduced movements can be a sign that Baby is in distress – so it is important to be aware of them.

Mum

Physically, this stage of pregnancy can be tough on Mum. She may be experiencing heartburn, constipation, wind, piles, cramps, breathlessness and dizziness. As the skin on her stomach continues to stretch, it may become itchy. She may be getting tired more easily again now and need to rest or nap more. She may also start to experience some discomfort when walking. However, if she is suffering from pain in the pelvic area, see pages 52–55.

Braxton Hicks contractions can become noticeable during the third trimester. These are just practice contractions, but sometimes they can be quite confusing for parents. Keep the section on birth handy (especially chapters 6 and 10), so that you are not making trips to the hospital only to find out that it is 'false' labour.

No laughing matter is Mum's need to visit the ladies' room in the later stages of pregnancy! As Baby grows, there is more pressure on her bladder, meaning frequent toilet stops or night-time awakenings. If Mum needs to go, she needs to go! Holding it can lead to over-tightening of the pelvic floor, which might put it into spasm and weaken it – this is not helpful for birth, where a strong pelvic floor will help Baby to rotate through the pelvis. So if you are out and about together and Mum says she needs to go, find her somewhere – and quickly!

As Baby takes up more room, Mum may experience a shortness of breath and increased tiredness. As you progress to the last few weeks you may see Mum's increased tiredness and then a sudden change – as if she has been energised. This will happen if the baby's head starts to descend into the birth canal and there is more space for her organs.

There is one last physical change that always amuses me: if Mum has an 'innie' belly button, towards the end of the pregnancy it is likely to become an 'outie' – this is perfectly normal and is not permanent.

Emotionally the third trimester can be one of the hardest for Mum, so again you need to be supportive and aware of the changes that are taking place. Mum will probably start to dream and fantasise about the baby from the start of the third trimester. It is also around the beginning of the third trimester that mums tend to start thinking about the labour and birth, which for some can lead to anxiety. Some mums may also develop an almost obsessive fear that their waters will break while they are out in public. By now you are getting the picture of the importance of your role to be a calm, reassuring presence, accepting all her concerns and fears as being real and not dismissing or ridiculing any of them. To Mum they are all very, very real.

Towards the middle and end of the third trimester is a period where mums can start to feel unattractive as the bump grows even bigger. Do your best to reassure her and do little things to show how much you love her.

Late on in third trimester you may experience the joys of a 'nesting Mum' – you might find your home cleaned and reorganised, you are likely to be required to finish all those jobs you 'haven't got around to yet' and she may even decide to redecorate.

Dad

Your fears and worries will start to surface during the latter stages of the pregnancy. It's important to confront these (see chapter 3 for more on this). You may also find yourself literally bouncing between the extremes of sheer joy and excitement to fear and trepidation. At work you are likely to start being distracted; now is not the time to be taking on important projects if you can avoid it. Try to enjoy these final stages because before long your child will be joining you and a whole new journey will begin.

Milestone

The big milestone in the third trimester is obviously the birth! Remember that it is quite normal for this to happen at any time between 37 and 42 weeks. Although you will have been given a due date, this is only an estimate, and only 5 per cent of babies arrive on theirs. A couple of weeks either side is normal!

A really good tip is, on the estimated due date (EDD), have something definite planned to do with your partner. It is very common for expectant mums to feel a little down if nothing has happened by the time the due date has arrived (and as you can see, the odds are that it won't have done). Take her out somewhere nice – to the cinema or for lunch. Make the due date an occasion where she gets a nice treat.

CHAPTER 2

Being a dad starts *here!*

So your partner has had the positive pregnancy test; you've possibly even attended a scan or two. Think there isn't much you can do until the baby gets here? Think that you haven't actually *become* a dad yet? Actually, this is one of the biggest myths of all. The truth is that you can make both labour and the early days with your newborn easier by being fully involved during the pregnancy.

Often dads refer to 'becoming a father' on the day their child is born. My own discussions and surveys with men show that this is a common feeling. On an emotional and psychological level, us blokes tend to be anything up to a full nine months behind our partners – not really fully bonding with our babies or seeing ourselves as fathers until the birth actually happens. This is understandable, really. Mums go through so many physical and emotional changes during pregnancy, whereas for us men, things often pretty much stay the same. This means that to be involved we need to make more of an effort. I refer to this process as 'antenatal bonding'. If your partner is pregnant and you are not feeling connected to your baby yet, don't panic, but do make the conscious decision to bond with your baby before she is born. Antenatal bonding for most of us men is not a natural process; it takes a conscious decision and effort to do it, but it has a massive impact on the bonding process – for both you and your baby.

Bonding with your baby

You affect your baby's development from the moment she is conceived. That's right, dads! Your attitude and support through-out pregnancy can directly affect how your baby grows and develops in the uterus. An awesome thought isn't it? Dr David Chamberlain, a renowned psychologist who has researched pre-natal development, psychology and bonding, refers to the time Baby spends in the womb as 'an intense learning period in one's life and time to establish patterns for a life-time'. That sounds pretty mind-blowing, but how does it happen?

Well, your unborn baby has ears by just three weeks (so probably before you even know you are expecting!). The ears are functional by 16 weeks and at 24 weeks Baby can hear sounds from outside. Some psychologists point to evidence of babies in the uterus being able to kick in time to music at 25 weeks! This means that for most of the pregnancy, your baby can hear your voice. She will know who you are and she will *already be bonding with you.*

This learning also forms the building blocks for what hap-pens postnatally. Once Baby is born, when you talk to her, she will recognise and respond to your voice from the times she heard it during pregnancy. Therefore, obviously the more she has heard you during pregnancy, once she is here your voice will be more familiar to her. This is brilliant in terms of being able to calm her when she arrives – you can almost see it as putting in time now with your baby, to allow her to get to know you. This will make it easier for you to calm and soothe her when she is here in your arms.

Why does bonding matter?

There is no one single reason why bonding with your unborn baby is important. In fact there are several pretty crucial ones, including:

■ **For your baby's development.** Helping to create a calm and positive environment is integral to the physiological development of your unborn baby. Any stress that Mum might feel during pregnancy increases the production of stress hormones, which can easily cross the placenta to the unborn baby. In moderation, these are beneficial to Baby's neurological development, but in excess they can have an adverse effect. So your role in creating a calm, stable home environment is important, from the start of pregnancy onwards.

■ **For your baby's wellbeing.** In order to ensure the healthiest outcome for your baby it is important to know her from the start. You may think your task is done now you've created the baby, but your job is only just beginning!

■ **For your own confidence.** Antenatal bonding is also important for your own confidence. You will find that the more connected you feel to your baby during pregnancy, the more you will be comfortable and at ease with your newborn when she arrives. Your baby will also sense this inner confidence and feel more secure and safe with you as a result, which again will help to keep her calm and bonded with you when she has arrived.

■ **For your relationship.** For you as a couple, life will feel more harmonious if you are putting in the time, effort and interest to make it so. Showing an interest in your baby and the pregnancy will help you to be closer to your partner, as she will feel that you value both her and the baby. Sometimes the pregnancy and postnatal days can be tough on couple relationships, so you valuing her is really important for creating and maintaining a strong foundation. For those of you who have chosen to breastfeed, evidence shows that involved dads lead to more successful breastfeeding, and breastfeeding is known for its positive health benefits for both Mum and Baby (for more on this, see chapter 15).

■ **For your own wellbeing.** It is finally becoming accepted that fathers, too, can suffer from postnatal depression (PND), and antenatal bonding can also help reduce the chances of it taking root in the first place. A common cause for PND in men is that they experience guilt when they don't instantly feel bonded with their baby. To compound this further, men can end up feeling excluded and isolated in their own family – because they are not bonded they retreat, becoming less and less involved with the baby, thus making their bonding issue worse. These are feelings where being proactive is a really positive way of preventing PND. Some men are fortunate to feel an instant bond with Baby at birth, but for many that bond establishes over time. It is harder for the bond to establish among all the additional pressures of becoming a family, so why leave it until the birth to start bonding with your child when you can start during the pregnancy?

'I knew we were pregnant, but it didn't really compute until that first scan. Then it became very real for me. It was pretty amazing, actually, which I hadn't expected. Seeing our baby on the screen and getting that scan photo meant it was really happening and gave me something to focus on. I couldn't wait for the next scan!' – **Matt**

case study

Okay, bonding is important ... so how do I do it?

There are some very simple things you can do to bond with your baby. I've provided a list of suggestions here. You *don't* need to do them all. Just choose those you feel comfortable with, but make the decision to *do something*.

1 If you have pictures from a scan, keep them to hand and look at them more often than just the one time at the scan visit! This will help you start to visualise your baby. As men, we find it hard to attach to things we can't see, hear or touch. This will help you start to think of your baby as a real person and start the bonding process.

2 Try greeting 'the bump' or your baby *as well as* your partner after coming home from work or an outing. You don't have to be over the top; a quick 'Hello, Baby' and a gentle pat on the bump is all it needs. Your baby will be able to hear and feel you!

3 Give your baby a name – this will make her more of a real person. It doesn't have to be the name she will actually have when she is born – it can just be a nickname.

4 Spend time together as a family. Talk, sing or play music to your baby, or maybe recite a rhyme or read a short story. Ideally choose one thing and repeat it each time. Your unborn baby will start to recognise a song, rhyme or story if she hears it repeatedly. Mums often say that their babies recognise particular CDs or a TV show theme song when they are born that they heard a lot during pregnancy! What is really great about this is not that your baby will recognise the story or song, but she will connect it to a time of feeling loved and content, and so, once born, singing this song or reading the same story is a great calming method for her.

5 At around 20–24 weeks you will be able to feel your baby move or kick. This is a great opportunity to become physically connected and bonded to Baby. Take time to feel her movements and as the pregnancy progresses you may want to try out some games, for example, some babies love playing hide-and-seek with Dad!

6 Start a blog. Daddy blogs are becoming popular – see my essential daddy blogs list at the end of the book (page 224) to get some ideas. You can record details about the scans or appointments, how you are both feeling or specific milestones. This will all help reinforce the fact that your baby is another person in the family already, and such records are great to look back on as Baby gets older.

'The pregnancy just didn't seem that real to me. Obviously I knew my partner was growing our baby in there, but I didn't feel particularly connected to him. I was just waiting until he was born, as I didn't think that I could bond with him until then. When I learnt about the benefits of bonding during pregnancy I thought it was something I should give a go to. I felt a bit stupid just talking or reading to the bump (it's just not *me*), but I play guitar, so I started to play my music for Baby, which felt a lot more natural. It did help and when our son arrived, he would happily listen to me play, so I think he remembered it!' – **David**

case study

Get involved – check your baby's movements

A baby's movements are an excellent indicator of her wellbeing and are a great bonding opportunity. As your baby develops, her number and type of movements will change with her activity pattern. She will have sleep periods that usually last between 20 and 40 minutes and rarely longer than 90 minutes

– something you could practise in preparation for the new-born days! The number of movements tends to increase until 32 weeks of pregnancy and then remain about the same, although the type of movement may change as the due date approaches. It is important to remember that babies should not stop moving towards the end of pregnancy and will continue to move right up until labour and often during birth.

While your partner may complain that her ribs have become a punch bag and her bladder is being used as a football, this is a great sign that your baby is well. You may, however, find yourself on the receiving end of a sharp tongue if you choose this moment to point this out! There are constructive ways you can help and be involved.

If your partner has had a busy day she may not have noticed the baby moving. Having a time when you can sit movement and bond with your baby. You can also orchestrate opportunities for Mum to feel the baby move herself – babies tend to move around more when she is resting. Run her a bath, bring her some chocolate, a cold drink or generally give her the chance to put her feet up and feel the baby kick, flutter, swish and roll!

If your partner ever feels uneasy about the pattern of movement, lack of movement or has any bad feelings about movement, encourage her to follow her instincts and contact her midwife or hospital. Mums know best! Never ignore a change of movements or allow her to go to sleep following a spell of reduced or erratic movements. Always encourage her to call her midwife or go to the hospital to be checked out.

You should also remember to be sympathetic to any discomfort your partner feels when the baby is kicking – after all you could be on the receiving end of her kicks for years to come!

For more information on movements during pregnancy visit www.countthekicks.org.uk.

So to sum up ...

There you go: no more 'There is nothing I can do to bond with my baby until she is here' or 'I'm not a dad yet'. You *are* now a dad and there are lots of things you can be doing, with huge benefits for you, your partner and your baby. It is worth the effort, so ask yourself, what are you going to do *today* to bond with your baby?

CHAPTER 3

What are you afraid of?

Come on guys, admit it … since you found out you are going to be a dad (or if you've taken on board my earlier point – see page 25 – you've found out that you're *already* a dad), you have had all sorts of thoughts and fears going around in your brain! Don't worry, this is totally normal and most of us guys go through the same. However, while it is completely normal to have these feelings, it's very important to try to understand and overcome them as much as you can.

Why is it so important to deal with fear?

The release of fear is a very important part of your preparation for both fatherhood and being a birth partner. It is particularly essential that you deal with any fears, as your anxiety can produce adrenalin in Mum – potentially leading to a prolonged or even stalled labour. I'll be explaining this more fully in chapter 7. Furthermore, if some fears are not dealt with, they can linger post-birth, causing tension, resentment and delayed bonding with your baby.

So what are common male fears?

Guys, listen up! These are the common ones, but in no way is this list exhaustive.

Who's the daddy?

First for the bombshell: research has shown up to six out of ten expectant fathers at some point in the pregnancy will suffer doubts and fears regarding the paternity of the unborn baby. On every course I teach, at least a couple of blokes have been, or are, dealing with this. It is so common, yet it is often not spoken about. This is an important fear to address because it can affect your behaviour during pregnancy, your attitude at the birth and your relationship with your baby.

If this thought has even fleetingly crossed your mind, I want you to now learn the likely reason for having it, then accept it and get rid of it! The reason for thinking this, in 99 per cent of cases, has absolutely nothing to do with the fidelity of your partner. It stems from the perfectly normal fears and anxieties you are having about fatherhood – and it manifests itself as this thought. It can be because you are in shock about your own ability to have achieved the miracle of creating a new life. Maybe you are in denial because you don't feel ready to be a dad.

Maybe you have had concerns about your own fertility. Maybe the baby was not planned and it was a bit of a surprise to you both. The list goes on, but the pattern is clear; it is solely linked to Dad's self-doubt and it is not to do with your partner.

Fortunately, for most men who have this thought, it is fleeting, and they are able to move on. For some, though, it sticks. They obsess about it and the thought can be extremely destructive. This is why you need to acknowledge that it is about you, not your partner – then deal with it and leave it behind. If this thought does continue to plague you despite your attempts to get past it, then it might be helpful to speak to a counsellor to try to resolve the underlying issue.

Money, money, money

We men also commonly worry about how our family will cope financially – that's the evolutionary inbuilt hunter–gatherer instinct kicking in! I am convinced, though, that if we all waited until we were in the right financial position to have children, humankind would be in danger of extinction! There is *never* a right time; whatever your situation *you can find a way* to manage.

Being hands-on

A very common anxiety is about actually handling a baby, being a bit heavy-handed or not knowing what to do. If you are worried about this, then do something about it! Take control and prepare yourself, attend good-quality antenatal education classes, which will give you a chance to learn the skills and practise them in advance. Check the resources section (see page 221) for recommendations. Spend time with friends or family who do have children. Remember one thing, though: you *will* learn what to do and if you put a little effort in, you will do just fine. Once your baby has arrived, it is normal to be a bit nervous at first, but practice makes a huge difference, so be a hands-on dad and get involved right from the very start.

Two becomes three

Men often worry about their relationship with their partner changing. Nope, sorry, I'm not going to tell you 'Don't worry it will hardly change' – and anyone who says that is talking ****. Yes, your relationship is going to change and, probably, quite dramatically. If this is your first baby, then you are no longer a couple; you are now a family. So allow yourselves both some time to adjust to this. In the early days and weeks, there is the possibility of you feeling like a spare part – unless you get actively get involved and get hands-on with dirty nappies and all!

The birth itself

Some of us are petrified at the thought of the birth and some will even feel physically sick. Again, this is not as unusual as you may think, and through preparation and understanding, for the majority of dads this fear can be eliminated. For some, though, the fear might remain, no matter how much effort they put into preparation. If this is the case, then you have to question whether you should really be there at the birth or, at the very least, whether you should be the main birth partner. You do have a choice. You could see whether there is a close family member or friend you would both feel comfortable with who would support you at the birth, or see whether you can find and afford a doula you both like (a doula is a birth professional who can offer you and your partner extra support during the labour and birth). I cover this all in more detail in chapter 7, so keep reading.

Not getting to the hospital on time

This worry is a big one with dads: 'What if we don't get to the midwife on time and I have to catch the baby?' This really does not happen that often – trust me. It is more likely that you *will* get to the hospital in plenty of time. However, it's a good idea to prepare yourself with the knowledge for how to cope if this rare event does happen. I cover this topic on pages 136–37, so if the unexpected does occur, you don't need to panic.

Whatever your fear, whether it is on this list or not, it is important to acknowledge it. There is no place for macho behaviour here. Failure to acknowledge that you have a fear and deal with it can have a big impact on your family. If you need additional support to cope with something that worries you, go to an antenatal class, talk to a midwife, email me, but *do something*. Don't let fear spoil the most amazing thing you are ever going to experience in your life.

CHAPTER 4

Sex in pregnancy

So the deed you did to get into this position in the first place can become a topic for confusion during pregnancy. Is it okay to keep on having sex? Will she want to? Will I want to? Can it hurt the baby?

Hormones and feelings

We are often told that women go through a cycle during pregnancy – first they go off sex, then they want it and then they go off it again. I have even seen a reference made to this period where pregnant women want it as them being likened to nymphomaniacs!

Of course, this may be true for some women, as the hormone changes may affect them in this way, but this is not a general rule. How they feel about sex may change from day to day, or they may well have an increased or decreased sex drive for the whole nine months. As well as the hormones, it's also going to depend on how she feels. In reality, Mum may well not feel up for sex if she is spending most of her day being sick – this is pretty understandable!

Many of women's biggest difficulties can be dealing with the changes in the body, which may now feel out of control. Some of these things will also feel deeply unattractive – big tummy, boobs leaking milk, stretch marks, heartburn and reflux, sickness – none of these things is a recipe for feeling sexy. While to you, she may still look perfect, if she doesn't feel that way herself it may well affect her libido.

'Sex was the last thing on my mind during the first trimester, when I just felt tired and sick all the time! It (my sex drive) did come back, though, when I started feeling a bit more like myself. Once the bump was big, though, we had to be a bit more inventive!' — **Melanie**

case study

Generally, I would suggest going into this one with a 'wait and see' attitude. Just as we all have different sex lives and drives before we get pregnant, we are not going to subscribe to a generalised pattern all of sudden just because we are having a baby. I don't think setting expectations is actually helpful to either us men or to women. Pregnancy is a period of adjustment for both Mum and Dad, and especially for first-time parents. It is the time we are likely to see some changes to our relationships. For us dads, if we have been led to have an expectation that during the second trimester our partner is going to suddenly be demanding sex night and day, we might actually start to worry unnecessarily if that doesn't happen ... which can lead us to feeling that maybe there is something wrong in our relationship, increasing potential friction and stress at what couldn't be a more delicate time.

Make sure you have time for just cuddles and affection – this is just as important as sex for keeping your relationship strong

'Pregnancy didn't do much for my libido. I went off sex for pretty much the whole nine months, and for a while after the birth too ...' – **Sally**

case study

and showing her that your feelings for her have not changed. But that's not all!

Just as importantly, though, it might be us who feel different about sex during pregnancy. Some women do rediscover their sex drive in the second trimester, only for us dads to be the ones who have totally lost ours.

It is not unusual for dads to go off sex during pregnancy and this can be for a number of reasons:

- For some of us, the sheer thought of having sex and placing our appendages near to our babies is enough for us to go off sex completely during pregnancy. Even though the truth of the matter is – and, trust me, I don't care how well-endowed you think you are – you will not be getting anywhere near to your baby. You will not hurt your baby and your baby will not be aware of what's going on.
- Some of us worry about hurting our partners, or have heard that sex can bring on premature labour. However, the idea that intense orgasms can bring on labour is a myth. There are times when sex is not advisable, such as if you have previously experienced miscarriage, or if pre-eclampsia has been diagnosed, but you will get guidance from your midwife or doctor in these situations.

■ For some of us, once our partner starts to look pregnant, we see her differently. She stops being our lover and gains an almost 'goddess-like' status – as the mother of our child she is there to just be revered. At this point sex is the last thing on our minds as we feel simply unworthy.

'When Jenny was more heavily pregnant it made me a bit nervous about harming the baby or causing her to go into labour! I wasn't expecting to feel like that, but I did, and even though I know it wasn't the case, I couldn't quite shake the idea, so sex became a lot less frequent.' – **Dan**

case study

On a practical level, if you are having sex during the pregnancy, as time goes by you may have to become a little more creative. The missionary position is not that advisable after about 20 weeks because you want to avoid squashing the bump and it's not good for Mum's circulation to spend time lying on her back. Of course, once Baby has arrived, all this sex business changes again. However, you have enough on your plate at the moment, so more on that later ...

CHAPTER 5

Pregnancy difficulties and complications

Every pregnancy is different. Some women glide through it, feeling wonderful and enjoying every moment ... in which case just skip this chapter! However, many women encounter some less-than-welcome symptoms as part of their experience. In this chapter, I've given you the lowdown on some of the key issues, and top tips for how to help if your partner experiences these. Don't worry about reading up on all the potential difficulties; just dip in and out of the sections that are relevant to your partner – if and when they occur.

The most common problems

Tiredness and fatigue

There is no one thing that has been proven to be the reason for pregnancy tiredness and fatigue, but with all the changes taking place in your partner's body, is it any surprise that she is likely to be feeling a little more tired than usual? Some have even compared the physical demands of pregnancy to running a marathon every day – it's tiring to even think about it.

So what is actually happening?

At the start of pregnancy, your partner's body has to effectively grow everything the baby needs, from producing the amniotic sac to the umbilical cord and placenta. Tiredness can be at its most profound even before your partner is showing the physical signs of her pregnancy, or even before she knows she is pregnant. Later in the pregnancy, as the baby grows, then so, too, do the additional demands for sustenance.

Nature always gives priority to Baby over Mum's needs, in respect of vitamins, energy and nourishment, so if Mum is not taking in enough of these to supply both herself and Baby, her needs may not be met. Add to that the increased hormone production, the gamut of emotions Mum is now going through, possible sleeplessness and morning sickness, it is no surprise that many women find pregnancy draining and even debilitating. So again, dads, you need to be there to recognise the signs and make sure you support Mum and your baby.

What can you and Mum do about tiredness?

Pregnancy tiredness or fatigue is normal, but by following these steps you can minimise the effect it has on your partner and baby.

- **Be aware of changes.** First off, you can make sure that you are aware of changes in your partner's general health and wellbeing – and Mum needs to accept that if she is tired, then she needs to rest. Remind Mum not to over-exert herself. Do things at an even pace and decide together to prioritise what is important to exert energy on and what is not. For very active women this can, of course, be very hard, and such mums need to learn how to relax. Attending a pregnancy yoga class or another relaxation method may be beneficial. As I have described earlier (see page 27), stress hormones in excess are not good for Baby's development.

- **Ask for help.** Don't be afraid to ask others for help. Your partner needs to know that she can ask you to do things for her and you both need to realise that it's okay to ask for help from friends and relatives. There is nothing wrong with asking other people to help you do the shopping, or to give you a hand if you have other children to collect from school or nursery. Keeping energy levels up may allow Mum to do other things that are good for her, like going for a walk in the fresh air to relax. This can have the benefit of assisting sleep at a time when getting good-quality sleep can be a bit of a struggle.

- **Take it easy.** While I'm talking about sleep, Mum should sleep as much as she feels she needs to. She may want naps during the day, especially as the pregnancy progresses. She may find staying up late for nights out becomes increasingly difficult, so don't let her feel pressurised into going to social situations when she does not feel like it. As my wife still reminds me to this day, 'During pregnancy, when women say they are tired, they mean *exhausted!*'

- **Watch your diet.** Diet is another massively important part of any pregnancy and it is vital to keeping Mum's energy levels raised as high as possible. Therefore work together to try to adjust both your diets to include plenty of protein and carbs. Remember that this should be a joint effort, but don't nag her about altering her diet. It is much better to support her by joining her in making dietary changes yourself and taking care of cooking some of the meals yourself (if you do not already do this). Calorific content is also important. Avoiding things such as chocolate and caffeine can be helpful; although these may give a quick energy boost the effects are short-lived, so Mum's energy levels can come crashing back down again. This can actually have the effect of making her more tired than before.

Eating little and often is a good way to keep energy levels up. It's also really helpful as the baby grows since there is less room available in the abdomen for the digestive system, so smaller meals are literally easier to stomach! Try encouraging Mum to get into the habit of eating little and often, six or seven times a day, as this will certainly help her feel less fatigued.

Now this will seem to fly in the face of everything I have said previously about resting and sleeping, but a cure for fatigue is *not* for Mum to become a couch potato. The right level of proper exercise can actually be invigorating. So make the most of the opportunity to do this together, which is also good for your relationship at this time of change. Find some nice walking spots, such as a local country park. Remember, though, that the aim is to rejuvenate Mum and not to wear her out, so keep the walks short and *don't overdo* it.

Sickness

Morning sickness affects over half of all pregnant women and for some it can be quite debilitating. Contrary to its name, 'morning' sickness can affect women at any time of day or night. For most it will cease at around the 12-week stage of pregnancy. One theory is that it is a natural reaction to the smells of food that may contain toxins harmful to the baby, therefore causing sickness to expel them. This is also believed to be why sickness subsides at 12 weeks for most women, as by then the baby is better able to defend itself against toxins.

It is also helpful for you to be aware that there is a link between stress levels and digestive issues, which can lead to stronger or prolonged episodes of sickness.

So how can you help calm morning sickness?
There are plenty of different suggestions for dealing with morning sickness. None of them is a cure, but for some women they may help lessen the symptoms of sickness.

- **De-stress.** Be aware of stressors in your partner's environment. Is there anything you can do to minimise potential stress?
- **Take control of the cooking for a while.** The associated smells of cooking food may trigger bouts of sickness. (See page 18 for information on foods to avoid that are not safe to eat during pregnancy.)
- **Reducing fibre and fat from the diet may help.** Try white bread instead of brown or cooked fruits rather than raw.
- **Encourage her to eat little and often.** This often helps and will also help to keep blood sugar levels more consistent.
- **Buy some lemons.** Smelling freshly cut lemons is thought to ease symptoms of sickness.
- **Stock up on ginger.** Ginger is often useful for its anti-nausea properties. Have it in the form of ginger tea, ginger biscuits or ginger sweets.
- **Keep snacks handy.** Store some dry crackers in the bedroom for when your partner first wakes in the morning, since eating first thing can help curb morning sickness.
- **Make some ice cubes.** If she is struggling to keep fluids down, make your partner some ice cubes so she can suck on them to help keep hydrated. You could even try adding some fruit juice to make them more exciting. Or buy her some lollipops to suck.
- **Buy her some acupressure wristbands.** She can use them to stimulate the 'Nei-Kuan' acupuncture point on her wrist. Some women say this really helps.
- **Keep breathing!** Encourage her to try deep-breathing exercises and relaxation techniques.

Hyperemesis gravidarum

Extreme sickness is referred to as *Hyperemesis gravidarum* and for a few women it can occur throughout the pregnancy. Dehydration is probably the greatest risk for women suffering from Hyperemesis. If your partner is constantly suffering from sickness, you need to make sure that she is taking in as much fluid as she can. If she is finding it difficult to hold down fluids, you should seek help from your GP. In extreme cases it may be necessary for your partner to be admitted to hospital for rehydration. *Do not ignore* extreme sickness or dismiss it as 'just part of being pregnant'. If you do see your GP and you feel the sickness is not being treated seriously, ask for a second opinion.

For more information and advice on *Hyperemesis gravidarum* see www.pregnancysicknesssupport.org.uk.

Hormone changes

Throughout the pregnancy Mum will experience a lot of hormone changes, which will affect her moods and her physical appearance. You should be aware of the possible effects of these hormone changes, as this will help your understanding and ability to work together through what can seem like strange occurrences!

Here is some information on the main hormones that will be surging through Mum's body during pregnancy:

- **Oestrogen.** One of the main hormones that change is oestrogen. This hormone is normally produced by the ovaries, but during pregnancy it changes to being produced by the placenta. By the end of the pregnancy, Mum's levels will be almost 100 times greater than before getting pregnant. The purpose of this increased oestrogen is to improve the blood supply by making just about everything grow, so obviously this is very beneficial for growing a baby! It also will cause others of Mum's body features to grow, from veins to moles, and it is also responsible for the breasts enlarging. The other effects of the increased oestrogen levels can include headaches, tiredness, cramps and mood swings.

■ **Progesterone.** Progesterone, like oestrogen, begins to be made by the placenta, and its production is controlled by the production of oestrogen. Progesterone works as a muscle relaxant and anti-inflammatory. It serves many purposes, including protecting the placenta and foetus from unwanted cells, suppressing contractions, as well as encouraging breast growth. Combined with oestrogen, while progesterone is in high levels it also prevents the production of breast milk. These levels plummet at the birth to allow another hormone, called prolactin, to be produced, which will stimulate the production of milk.

Along with the oestrogen, increasing progesterone levels are one of the main reasons for Mum's mood swings.

■ **Prolactin.** During pregnancy prolactin is also partly responsible for the growth of the mammary tissue and those enlarging breasts. Prolactin comes into its own when the oestrogen and progesterone levels drop off. Its production is the combined effect of thyroid and insulin and is essential for the production of breast milk.

There are plenty of other hormone changes that occur, but there are other places where you can find this information, so I will leave it there. Save to say that while there isn't much you can do to lessen the symptoms of surging hormones, understanding their role in the pregnancy and the fact that your partner may not be in complete control of her moods or emotions, just might give you a little more understanding and help you to safely navigate your way through!

Swelling (oedema)
Swelling is extremely common in pregnancy and is thought to affect nearly half of all pregnant women. Mums may experience swelling around their fingers, ankles, face or even lower back. This is more likely to happen in the last few months.

Swelling is usually caused by two factors. The first is water retention, which is thought to be Nature's way of ensuring that Mum stays hydrated so that Baby has access to enough fluids. Second is the increased volume of blood in Mum's body, adding to pressure on the veins in the legs and also major arteries and veins in the groin.

Normally the swelling will get progressively worse as the day goes on, as these fluids are affected by gravity and drain down to the feet and hands. Time of year can also have a marked impact on swelling and your partner is more likely to suffer during periods of hot weather. Again, rest is important since tiredness has also been linked with increased swelling.

Now, although swelling is normal, the symptoms should not be ignored as they could suggest other possible complications. So it is important that you both keep an eye on the symptoms and if you are in any doubt, contact your midwife or GP.

The main signs to be concerned about are:

■ **If the swelling is not just localised at the ankle** but starts to travel up the calf. Try pressing on the swelling – if the dent remains, it is a possible sign of pre-eclampsia (see page 57). Pre-eclampsia can lead to more serious complications, so if you are at all concerned, you should seek medical advice straight away.

■ **If the swelling comes on suddenly or very noticeably** in the hands, face or feet – again this could be a possible sign of pre-eclampsia, so you should also seek advice urgently.

■ **If the swelling occurs just in one leg,** you should check the calf – if it is tender, lumpy or even red it could be a blood clot, so you should seek medical advice as soon as possible.

■ **If your partner's hands and wrists are swollen.** This could be a sign of carpal tunnel syndrome, when the swelling may be pressing on the nerves that are in the arm and can lead to a tingling sensation or feeling of numbness as the nerves are affected. Seeking medical help is important as carpal tunnel syndrome needs to be managed to help ensure that there is no permanent damage to the nerves in the wrists.

What can you do to help?

Although it may not be possible to prevent some swelling from developing, there are things you can both do to minimise its occurrence. It is important to try to support your partner to do this since severe swelling can make her legs very painful, but also her skin sensitive to touch.

As with most pregnancy conditions, diet can play a very important part. Eating a balanced diet is important, and it is beneficial to try to make sure that Mum gets an element of protein in each meal.

Make sure Mum is getting her five-a-day and also try to help her reduce her intake of foods with high salt, fat or sugar content. Help her avoid eating ready meals or processed foods as these normally contain quite high levels of salt and other ingredients and these can worsen fluid retention. Most meats we buy now contain high levels of water, and additives are used to retain the water, so be selective about the meats you buy. Vitamins C and E are great for pregnant women, so try to help her increase her consumption of those foodstuffs that naturally contain them.

Vitamin C boosters

To gain a boost of vitamin C, try:

- Peppers, both red and green.
- Melons.
- Strawberries (if in season).
- Potatoes.
- Tomatoes.
- Citrus fruits.
- Broccoli.
- Cabbage.

Vitamin E boosters

For vitamin E look to the following:

- Sunflower seeds.
- Sweet corn.
- Cooking or dressing in vegetable oils such as sunflower, corn or wheat germ.
- Nuts such as cashews and almonds. (There is conflicting advice about eating nuts during pregnancy, so make sure you follow the most up-to-date guidance available, which the midwife will discuss with Mum at her first appointment. If you are unsure about this, please consult your GP. Also be aware of nut allergies.)

Drinking water

Drinking lots of water is also important. I realise this may seem counterproductive if you are trying to avoid swelling, but trust me it isn't. There is no point in Mum thinking that she will cut down on fluid intake to try to alleviate the swelling, as this does not work. She needs to continue to keep her fluid intake up, as water will actually help the kidneys to filter the excess fluids.

To assist the function of the kidneys, some foods can have the effect of making Mum go to the toilet more, but this will also help. This always raises a smile with mums, as one of the common complaints is simply the number of times they are going to the toilet each day! Foods you can try to assist the kidney are apples, oranges, grapefruit and also foods such as celery and watercress. The intake of garlic is also thought to aid the circulation – so get plenty of that into your cooking!

What else can you do to help swelling?

- **Go shopping!** Take your partner out to buy her some new shoes. If her feet are swollen, her shoes will feel tight or not fit her at all. Some flat or very low-heeled shoes that will stretch to accommodate her swollen feet will be ideal – maybe even a size larger than she normally takes.

- **Encourage Mum to rest as much as possible.** Also when she is resting make sure that her feet are raised above the level of her hips. Find her a footstool or put a cushion on to the coffee table for her to use when she is sitting down.

- **While sitting she can do some foot exercises.** This encourages the fluid to drain away. She can try bending her feet up and down quickly 20 to 30 times on each side. Circling her feet first one way, then the other, for 10 rotations in each direction also works in the same way.

- **When Mum is sitting, encourage her to not cross her legs.** This can restrict the blood flow and encourage pooling. If Mum *has to* stand for any length of time, she should try shifting her weight from foot to foot, so that each foot is rested in turn.

- **If Mum is lying down**, encourage her to lie on her left-hand side. This will stop compression of the venae cavae (the major veins that return blood flow to the heart from the limbs) and keep the blood circulating, supporting fluid drainage. When sleeping it can also help to raise the lower end of the mattress by popping a pillow underneath the feet – so that gravity can drain fluids from the feet and ankles overnight.

- **Become Mum's private masseur!** Dads, now's your chance! You can offer practical help by giving Mum a foot and leg massage. Use a pregnancy oil and gently stroke from her feet upwards (imagine you are stroking all that fluid up her legs, away from the feet). Depending on the level of swelling, this may be uncomfortable. If it is – stop. Just remember, when using any oils, make sure that you test a little bit on an area of skin and leave for 30 minutes before massaging, just to make sure that Mum doesn't have an adverse reaction to it.

- **How about some cabbage leaves?** Something to try if Mum is getting very desperate: cabbage leaves. Cabbage is thought to draw out surplus fluids and so can ease the discomfort. Get some nice big fresh leaves, give them a quick wipe but don't wash them, and then place them on any areas that seem swollen. You can keep some leaves in the fridge to add a relieving, cooling effect. Wrap them around the swollen areas. You will find that the leaves will become wet to touch – when they do, change them for fresh ones. You can do this as often as Mum wants.
- **Have a nice herbal cuppa!** Now many mums will experiment with herbal teas during pregnancy. A great one to try for swelling is dandelion tea. This is thought to possibly help with fluid retention. Always read the guidance on any herbal teas before drinking them (you will usually find this on the packet), though there may be conditions under which they should not be used and some are not suitable for use during pregnancy.

Once Baby is here, it is worth you being aware that Mum is quite likely to find that the swelling will become even worse in the few days following the birth. This is simply as Mum's body readjusts. All the extra blood, tissues and fluids needed during the pregnancy must now be broken down and got rid of. This is a temporary cycle – as Mum goes to the loo over the first few days this will help that pass.

Symphysis Pubis Dysfunction (SPD) and Pelvic Girdle Pain (PGP)

I am always surprised at the number of pregnancy books that do not cover a condition that is thought to affect one in four of all pregnant women: SPD.

SPD is a condition often associated with pregnancy. Its symptoms can also persist after the birth of the baby and in some women it can be quite debilitating. It can occur at any stage during the pregnancy and can affect all pregnant women, although it is more likely to occur in those who have babies quite close together. It is also related to another pregnancy condition called pelvic girdle pain (PGP) and often the two conditions are even referred to as being the same thing. Up to 7 or 8 per cent of women continue to suffer the symptoms after the birth of their baby.

So what is it? Basically the condition causes excessive movement of the pubic symphysis, which is a stiff joint at the front of the pelvis, causing a misalignment of the pelvis. Your partner's body will produce a hormone called relaxin, which will soften the supporting ligaments, so in some cases they are unable to properly support the pelvis. It is necessary for the body to soften the ligaments so that the pelvis can stretch and make room to birth your baby, but for some women the pelvic joints move more during and just after pregnancy, causing inflammation and pain.

Walking can become difficult and painful, and some women find it very problematic. Interestingly the condition has been known about for centuries, even as far back as Hippocrates, but it seems to have become more common in recent years. It is unknown whether this is simply because more women are reporting the symptoms or possibly because the average age of pregnant women is rising.

Signs that your partner may be suffering from SPD include:

- **A popping or clicking noise** when walking or move about.
- **Discomfort or pain in the pelvis.** This pain will normally be emanating from the front of the pelvis.
- **Pain in the hips,** groin or bottom are also signs to look out for.
- **Your partner may walk with a waddle** and find it hard to lift things or climb stairs. She may also have difficulty standing or carrying out many other normal day-to-day activities.

■ **Your partner may show signs of antenatal depression.** Some people think that SPD causes antenatal depression, especially when the pain is extreme and prolonged, so it is important that the signs are spotted early and help sought.

It is also important to seek help early for SPD as this will minimise the effect in the medium to long term. Not all medical professionals are fully aware of the scope of this condition, so, dads, make sure you support your partner in getting the proper help without being brushed off with 'It's just a normal part of pregnancy'. Remember that you can always ask to be referred to a specialist or for a second opinion.

Unfortunately there is no research available on how to cure the condition, but if diagnosed your partner may be issued with crutches, a support belt or pain relief. Some women, if the waiting lists are not too great, will also be referred to a maternity physiotherapist to learn some exercises to help build strength – to protect the pelvis and prevent the condition worsening.

Other options include seeing a specialist osteopath or a reflexologist – who in different ways may be able to help your partner find some relief from her discomfort.

What should you do if your partner is suffering from SPD?

You certainly should take SPD into account when you are thinking about and writing your birth preferences (see chapter 8). Although often during labour women are not aware of the discomfort from SPD, it is still important to take care, especially when you are considering the positions for giving birth in. One of the best positions for your partner, if she is suffering from SPD or PGP, is a kneeling position (see page 68) – either upright or leaning forwards over a birth ball, a chair or the headboard of the bed. Before birth, she should explore the maximum width her legs can be apart without discomfort or pain and you should take note of this so she doesn't overextend during the birth. Therefore you will need to remind or tell the midwife/doctor that you have SPD/PGP. If you need to use stirrups for any reasons, these can potentially strain the pelvis further, causing long-term problems. If, for any reason, stirrups have to be used, then the legs should be moved to-gether very gently and slowly, in matching positions. This is extremely important since if Mum starts to worry and be fear-ful about moving or doing anything during labour that she knows is going to hurt she is likely to produce adrenalin, which, as you will read about in chapter 7 (see page 73), is what you should try to avoid at all costs.

During pregnancy, make sure you are always trying to minimise your partner's need to lift anything heavy. Many women find sitting on a birth ball the most comfortable way to sit, so you could buy her one of these to try out. Also invest in a good pregnancy pillow that she can use for sleeping, as these can help support and stabilise her pelvis while asleep. You can now buy specially designed pregnancy pillows that help you to lie on your left side and also keep your legs raised while you sleep.

Where possible, help her to avoid tasks such as hoovering, pushing buggies or manoeuvring supermarket trolleys around corners (as this action causes the pelvis to twist and place increased strain on it), standing for too long or any strenuous activity. Crossing legs also increases strain on the pelvis, and when getting in and out of a car or on or off a bed, she should swing her legs together – so keeping her knees and ankles together – as again this reduces strain on the pelvis.

For further help you can contact the Pelvic Partnership www.pelvicpartnership.org.uk.

Strep B infection

Group B Streptococcus (GBS or Group B Strep) is a very com-mon bacterium, carried normally, without harm or symptoms by up to 30 per cent of adults (both men and women), in the intestines and by up to 25 per cent of women in the vagina. Carrying it causes no problems or symptoms, but GBS can cause serious infections – typically pneumonia, septicaemia (blood poisoning) and meningitis – most commonly in babies around the time of birth and up to about three months of age. Most of these infections are preventable.

What can I do?

Make sure you and your partner know about GBS and about when a newborn baby is at raised risk of GBS infection. These are where Mum has:

- Previously had a baby with GBS infection.
- A vaginal or rectal swab taken during the current pregnancy, which grew GBS.
- GBS grown from a urine sample (she should be treated at the time of diagnosis) during the current pregnancy.
- A temperature of 37.8°C (100°F), or higher, during labour.
- Labour starting or waters breaking before 37 completed weeks of pregnancy.
- Waters breaking more than 18 hours before delivery.

If any of these situations apply to your partner, then she should be offered intravenous (via a vein) antibiotics from the start of labour and at intervals until the baby is delivered. This treatment is hugely effective at stopping GBS infections developing in newborn babies

Can my partner find out whether she carries GBS?

Yes. Testing for GBS is available privately, although most NHS hospitals in the UK don't offer it routinely, unlike some other countries. A positive GBS result is reliable, but the NHS tests are not very sensitive and only detect up to half of carriers.

Sensitive GBS tests are available privately, with home kits costing around £35 (see www.gbss.org.uk/test for where to get these).

Testing is best done at 35+ weeks of pregnancy since a sensitive test result is very predictive of GBS status for up to five weeks.

What next?
Testing isn't essential, but it is very important to know when a baby is at greater risk of developing Group B Strep infection and what action can minimise this risk. Be informed and ensure that your partner is too. For more information visit www.gbss.org.uk.

Pre-eclampsia
Pre-eclampsia usually develops during the third trimester – after 27 weeks of pregnancy have gone by. It can be very mild or range to severe. Mum might not be aware of the symptoms and feel perfectly healthy, so regular antenatal check-ups are important in order to detect the signs. Experts think that pre-eclampsia happens when the placenta is failing to function properly and if it is not treated effectively it can make Mum and Baby ill, sometimes seriously.

At every antenatal appointment, the midwife or doctor will do tests in order to search for any possible signs. This is why they check Mum's blood pressure and ask for a urine sample each time to see whether it contains protein.

Obviously, you and your partner won't be able to carry out these checks yourselves, but there are some other symptoms that you can keep an eye out for, including:

- Feeling generally out of sorts and unwell.
- Bad, sudden swelling in her face, hands or ankles, feet and legs.

- Bad headaches.
- Vomiting.
- Weight gain (because of fluid retention).
- Blurred vision or flashing before her eyes.
- Bad pain under her ribs.

Support and more information

If you have any concerns at all, in the first instance talk to your midwife or GP. For more information and support you can also contact Action on Pre-Eclampsia via http://action-on-pre-eclampsia.org.uk.

Ectopic pregnancy and miscarriage

Very sadly, in some circumstances a pregnancy will not survive. When a baby is lost before 24 weeks of pregnancy, this is called a 'miscarriage'.

Some fertilised eggs implant in the wrong place, especially in the fallopian tube, though they can happen in the ovary or cervix, instead of the uterus. Where a pregnancy develops outside the uterus, this is called an 'ectopic' pregnancy. As an ectopic pregnancy develops, it causes pain and bleeding and, left untreated, there is the risk of internal bleeding. This means that an ectopic pregnancy is a medical emergency and can be potentially life-threatening for the mum if it is not treated. If a pregnancy is ectopic, there is, sadly, no way that the pregnancy can survive.

What are the symptoms of a miscarriage?

The most obvious signs are period-like pains and heavy bleeding, which may include blood clots. However, it is possible to miscarry without being aware of it, especially early in pregnancy. Many women mistake a miscarriage for a late period, or sometimes the miscarriage may not be discovered until you have a scan. **If you have any concerns about a**

possible miscarriage, seek advice and support from a medical professional.

What are the symptoms of an ectopic pregnancy?

If there is any doubt at all, get advice from your midwife or GP. Symptoms to look out for include:

- **Unusual vaginal bleeding** that is different from a normal period (it may be lighter, brighter, darker red or more watery than usual).
- **Mild to severe pain**, usually on just one side, in the lower abdomen or pelvis.
- **Feeling light-headed**, faint or dizzy and perhaps sweating.
- **Diarrhoea** or pain during a bowel movement.
- **Going into shock or collapsing.** This is very serious, as it signifies severe internal bleeding and you should seek emergency medical help.
- **Pain at the tips of the shoulders**, which feels worse when she lies down. This happens if internal bleeding irritates other internal organs, such as the diaphragm.

There are different ways of treating a suspected ectopic pregnancy. If it is discovered early it can be treated with drugs; however, sometimes surgery may be necessary. If you are worried about a possible ectopic pregnancy, you should seek medical advice and support.

Coping after the loss of a pregnancy

The impact of losing a pregnancy can be hard for you both, as you each go through the emotions of loss. In some cases, and this is more likely with an ectopic pregnancy, Mum may also be physically recovering from surgery, and this can potentially have a knock-on impact upon her fertility. Make sure you support each other during this difficult time and, if you are finding it hard to cope, speak to a GP, health visitor or mental health professional for further help.

For more support on these issues, go to: the Ectopic Pregnancy Trust, www.ectopic.org.uk, or the Miscarriage Association, www.miscarriageassociation.org.uk.

Male pregnancy symptoms (Couvade Syndrome)

I cannot write a book like this without including this one, can I? It is now recognised that dads can be so in tune with their pregnant partners that they will display similar pregnancy symptoms. This can be anything from morning sickness or heartburn to even developing their own pregnancy 'bump' (no, I do *not* mean a beer belly!). The official name for this condition is Couvade Syndrome.

One theory is that Couvade Syndrome occurs due to hormonal changes occurring in the man – which is actually not that far-fetched. (You will read about the hormonal impact on us dads when we become fathers in the third section of this book – see page 195.) Some of these symptoms can be quite severe, so it's important to be aware that it can happen. Depending on the study, the percentage of men who experience Couvade Syndrome ranges widely – from 10 to 65 per cent. As with many things, the exact number is unknown, as many men may only experience mild symptoms, which they may not ever report. If this does happen to you, don't worry. But if you are concerned you can ask your GP for support, or alternatively contact me at DaddyNatal: dean@daddynatal.co.uk.

section two
Labour and birth

CHAPTER 6

The basics of labour and birth

Okay, dads, this chapter is a quick overview of the basics that you need to know about labour and birth, including some key terms that it's best to be familiar with upfront! The remaining chapters in this section will go into more detail on practical roles, tools and techniques that you can use during labour.

Labour

First up, you really need to know what labour is! Well it basically means the uterus working (or even labouring!) towards bringing your baby out into the world. What is the uterus? Well, this is the place where Baby spends nine months growing and developing and it's made up of muscle. Contractions are the movements of the muscle as it works towards getting your baby out.

At the bottom of the uterus is the cervix, which is closed during pregnancy to keep baby in and infection out, but during labour, the cervix will open.

The hormone that gets labour going and keeps it progressing is called oxytocin (pronounced 'oxy – toe – sin') and this is a good term to become familiar with as it will impress your other half! The basic idea is that you want as much oxytocin produced as possible during labour! However, the hormone that can stall labour and can make it a more painful and longer experience is called adrenalin, which is caused by fear, anxiety, fatigue and feeling uncomfortable, so it's important that your partner feels as relaxed as she can – and you can help her with this.

When might labour begin?

At your first scan (usually around 11–14 weeks) you will be given an Estimated Due Date (EDD). This is determined by a set of measurements taken at the 12-week scan. Due dates are notoriously inaccurate, as only 5 per cent of babies are actually born on theirs!

In fact, a normal term of pregnancy is between 37 and 42 weeks, so, with this in mind, it is helpful if you can avoid focusing on a single date, but to think about how it would be perfectly normal for the birth to happen any time in those few weeks. This also means that the pregnancy is not technically 'overdue' until you reach 42 weeks. In reality, labour begins when Mum's body and Baby are ready!

How do you know labour has begun?

There are signs that labour may have started, which include:

- Contractions.
- The amniotic fluid around the baby being released (known as the 'waters breaking').
- Mum has a bloody show (blood-stained mucus from the vagina).

However, it is also important to notice that Mum may experience these symptoms and it does not automatically mean that labour has started. A good example of this is Neil's story on pages 137–38), whose partner's waters broke a full week before she went into labour.

If you suspect that Mum's waters have broken, but there are no other signs of labour, it is a good idea to let your midwife know as soon as possible so that Mum and Baby can be checked to make sure all is okay. If you and your partner think the waters have broken and it is before 37 weeks of pregnancy, seek medical advice urgently.

How do you know where you are in labour?

Generally labour is divided into three phases or 'stages', which makes it a bit easier to work out roughly where you are, but as every stage of labour takes a different length of time for every woman, this doesn't really give you any idea as to how long you have to go!

Labour is usually medically defined in three parts:

■ **First stage** – where the uterus works to open the cervix.
■ **Second stage** – where the uterus works to birth the baby.
■ **Third stage** – where the uterus works to birth the placenta.

Let's break down each of these three parts into more detail:

The first stage

Just to complicate things a little for you – the first stage of labour is actually divided into two separate stages: 'pre' labour and 'active' labour.

Pre labour

At this point, the cervix will be dilating (opening) up to about 4 cm (by the time your partner is ready to give birth, it will have opened to around 10 cm). Mum is likely to be experiencing contractions and may feel that she is already working quite hard through them. However, medically this part of labour is called 'pre' labour. During this time contractions may be irregular. No two labours are ever the same and often this stage can last for several hours.

It is helpful to have discussed this stage of labour already and for Mum to have practised the different positions she may want to use, also to make sure you have included your preferred position on the birth plan (see page 89) in advance, to refer to. However, if on the day she feels more comfortable in a position you hadn't planned, then support her into that as it's hard to know ahead of time what will work best for you.

First stage – active labour

Pre labour then moves to what is known as 'active' labour, when the cervix's dilation has reached 4 cm and now is opening to 10 cm. Usually by this point the contractions have started to become more regular, closer together and longer-lasting. There is no way for you to examine the cervix to try to work out how far along she is (so don't even think about it!), but you can monitor her contractions to help gauge how she is progressing. It may be handy to jot them down in a notebook, as it's easy to lose track.

Transition

This point comes at the end of active labour, which some women experience, and is often referred to as 'transition'. Not all women experience transition, but many do, so it is helpful for you to know what to expect, just in case.

Transition occurs towards the very end of the first stage, so the good news is that if you spot your partner going through this, then the chances are you are not far off from meeting your baby! During transition there is a surge of adrenalin that floods Mum's body. This is all part of her body gearing up for birthing your baby, and part of something called the 'natural expulsive reflex'. Now don't worry at this point, this is 'good' adrenalin not the 'bad' stuff, so you don't need to be 'preventing' it – or trying to. However, for some women, this adrenalin surge will come with side effects, which can be a bit unsettling if you do not realise what they are. These symptoms can be physical or emotional. Physically, all that adrenalin can lead to Mum having the 'shakes' – jiggling legs or shivering is common. She might begin to feel very hot, or suddenly start feeling nauseous – or even like vomiting.

Emotionally, all that adrenalin can also send Mum into an emotional 'fight or flight', and is also often known as the 'self-doubt phase'. Even the calmest woman at this point may start suddenly saying 'I can't do it' or 'I want a Caesarean'. My wife, Steph, in both our hospital births, started to demand to go home at this point in labour!

Second stage – giving birth to your baby

During the second stage, contractions are now taking place to ease the baby out of the uterus and into your arms.

Some positions will make the birth easier and some will make it more difficult. Despite what you see on TV, if your partner is giving birth lying on her back, it is going to make the process more difficult, as it restricts available space in the pelvis and also means she is almost birthing against gravity. There is also an increased risk of perineal damage in this position (i.e. tearing of the skin around the vaginal opening), so for your partner's own comfort during and after the birth, this is one to avoid if possible.

Positions that can make this second stage a little easier for Mum include:

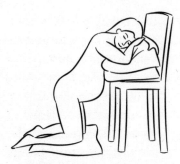

Kneeling against something

Being on all-fours

Lying on her side. (If Mum is tired and needs to lie down, being on her side will make the birthing easier than being on her back, but you may need to be called on to hold that leg up!)

The third stage – birthing the placenta

The placenta has grown during pregnancy and is what has nourished your baby throughout it. Now that the pregnancy has finished with the birth of your baby, the job of the placenta is done, so the body will expel it. This is the third stage of labour, and, if all has been straightforward during the birth, you will have a choice as to whether you birth the placenta naturally or medically.

Birthing the placenta 'naturally' means waiting for the body to start contractions again and then to birth it. Sometimes this happens very quickly, literally within minutes of the birth of the baby. Sometimes, however, it can take longer, although staying warm and allowing baby to try and breastfeed will help.

Birthing the placenta 'medically' means Mum receiving an injection in her thigh to stimulate contractions quickly. The benefits are that there is less likely to be bleeding immediately after the birth, but there is an increased risk of having to return to hospital because of bleeding later on, due to remnants of the placenta being left behind in the uterus. As with any injections, there is always the risk of Mum having an adverse reaction. If she has had a long or difficult labour, a medically managed third stage may be recommended because of the increased risk of heavy bleeding following the birth.

Caesarean section (or C-section)

Not all babies are born vaginally and around one in four arrives in this world via Caesarean section. There is evidence that suggests that with better support and education this rate could be hugely reduced, so getting prepared for your role in the birth is really important.

A Caesarean section is an operation and involves a cut being made through Mum's abdomen and uterus. This is usually performed under a spinal or epidural anaesthetic. In cases where the Caesarean is an emergency, or there are other medical/preferential reasons, they can be carried out under general anaesthesia.

Caesareans that are planned in advance are known as 'elective' or 'planned' Caesareans, while Caesareans that take place at short notice, usually during labour, are called 'emergency' Caesareans. This means many 'emergency' Caesareans are carried out for reasons not related to urgent medical emergency, but also for reasons such as labour having stalled.

While it can feel as though there isn't much you can do during a Caesarean, your role at a Caesarean birth is just as important, which I will cover in the next chapter. If you and your partner are planning a Caesarean birth in advance, you can still write a birth plan outlining your wishes for the birth, and I will look at this in the chapter on birth preferences (see page 109).

Birth preparation – especially for dads!

Now the rest of this section is going to really make you focus on your specific role in birth and how you can make this journey even easier. So keep reading to find out lots more.

Your role

The previous outline gives you an idea of what Mum's body is doing during labour, but what will *you* be doing to help her body achieve this? The following chapter will give you a practical insight to what you can be doing.

Writing a birth plan

It is crucial to write a birth plan (see chapter 8 for more on this), so that you *both* know what you are expecting from the birth, but also so that you have time to research all the different options available to you – including key choices such as where to have your baby, methods of pain relief you would like to learn about or have access to, your choices during and immediately after the third stage of labour. Chapter 11 will go into more detail about the kinds of interventions that might be offered before or during labour, how you can weigh up whether they are needed and if you and your partner feels comfortable with them.

CHAPTER 7

Dad's role during labour

What can Dad *do* during labour and birth?

This is the question I am probably asked the most by dads, and it is normally followed by a 'witty' comment from someone else such as 'mopping her brow' or worse 'keep out of the way!' These comments couldn't be further from the truth ... dads can do so *much* during labour and really make a difference. Unfortunately, no, I cannot guarantee that everything will go to plan; I cannot wave a magic wand and, no, we definitely can't swap places!

If I was to tell you that you have it within your power to affect the length of your partner's labour, the degree of pain she may or may not feel during labour, even the outcome of the birth – whether interventions are required or even whether she has a Caesarean section – how would you feel? Here is the newsflash – *it's all true*. So rather than making jokes about being a 'spare part' in the delivery room, dads should take responsibility for their role, accept and make sure they do everything they can to ensure that their impact on the birth is positive and not negative.

In fact, as I've mentioned before, it is this massive bearing on the progress and outcome of birth that led world-renowned Michel Odent, champion of natural childbirth and water-birthing, to argue that dads should not even be present at the birth. He even went as far as to blame nervous dads in the delivery room for the increase in Caesarean rates. At the time, many people were incensed by his comments, including myself, initially. In truth, though, I actually found that in a lot of respects I agreed with him – dads *can* have a negative impact on childbirth. The difference is that I don't think the answer is to simply remove dads from birth, because dads who are properly supported and informed can be the most excellent birth partners, with benefits that are far-ranging and crucial for the whole family.

In most cases, your partner will want you to be there at the birth of your child, as there is nobody she would rather have with her. You made this baby together, you are life companions, you bring her security and compassion, and now you are going to welcome your baby into the world together. But with this comes responsibility to understand what is going on and responsibility to be the best support you can be to her. Therefore preparation for a positive birth experience is *not* just the domain of the woman.

So if you want to be there, what can you do?

Your role in labour is really only about two things. So dads, listen up, *understand* your role, *prepare* for your role and really *support* your partner!

Role one: be her protector

Yep, you get to be her knight in shining armour! But what are you protecting? Everything in this role relates from one key factor – adrenalin.

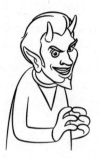

Adrenalin = the bad guy

Adrenalin is the enemy of labour and it is produced in the labouring woman if she becomes afraid or anxious. As her protector you are trying to help protect your partner from getting an attack of adrenalin!

When a woman is in labour her body creates a hormone called oxytocin (as mentioned on page 63). This hormone relaxes the woman and makes labour happen. However, the hormone adrenalin is the enemy of oxytocin. If adrenalin is produced it neutralises oxytocin and the labour stalls. This leads to contractions slowing and labour becomes more painful. The combination of both these factors can lead to interventions taking place to restart things, making it more likely that the birth will require assistance. By removing adrenalin from the picture (or preventing it ever being there in the first place) oxytocin can do its job and allow labour to progress.

Overleaf is a simple pictorial story, which will help you to remember this. It shows how and why adrenalin has this effect on labour.

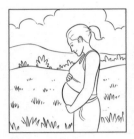

Woman is in labour.

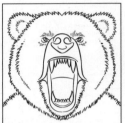

Woman sees a Grizzly Bear.

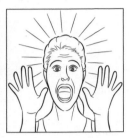

Woman's brain senses danger. Body produces adrenalin in response to seeing this threat.

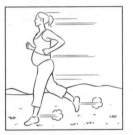

Adrenalin diverts blood flow from the uterus to heart, lungs and legs which stalls labour, and allows woman to scarper to place of safety.

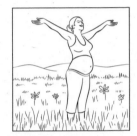

When woman has reached place of safety and relaxes again, adrenalin dissipates and oxytocin resumes labour.

What causes her to feel fear?

So your role as a protector is about protecting your partner's birthing environment and recognising and handling anything that may cause fear – the 'grizzlies in the room' – and allow that adrenalin to start pumping around her body. But what can cause this adrenalin to start? After all, you are fairly unlikely to run into a real grizzly bear in hospital!

The environment

Opposite is an image of a typical hospital delivery room. So, what in this room could cause an adrenalin surge? What could cause apprehension or fear in your partner?

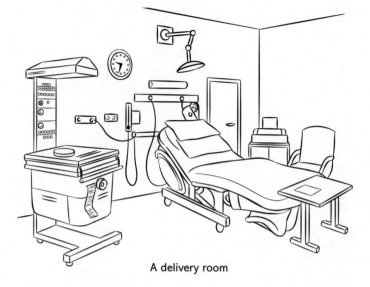

A delivery room

Simple: just about everything! Even the clock on the wall can cause both of you to watch time pass and worry about how long labour is taking. How about the blood pressure band hanging behind the bed? What about the alarm call button or the baby resuscitator? Maybe the IV tree sitting just at the head of the bed? All of these things can evoke anxiety in either of you, which can start the process of adrenalin production.

The most important thing to remember is: *don't panic!*

Simply by recognising that these things can cause anxiety is a first step. Now you are aware, you can talk about them, understand them and accept that they are there not for you, but simply because they are always there. If you spot something in your partner's eye line you feel may cause a problem, move it! Think about how you can play down the medicalised atmosphere of the delivery room, with dimmed lights or music playing.

These are tangibles that you can spot and deal with, but also think about the walk into the hospital, checking in, being examined. Just walking into the maternity suite can be scary, as it all becomes very real for both of you. Is it any surprise that many women, when arriving at hospital, will state that 'My contractions have slowed down'? That's caused by that surge of adrenalin neutralising the oxytocin. So be aware, once you get there make your partner as comfortable as possible and the environment as relaxing as possible, as quickly as possible. Reassure her and follow my labour dos and don'ts in chapter 12!

'We arrived at the hospital and suddenly the contractions really slowed down. I knew that this was probably because we had changed our environment and Catherine was having an adrenalin surge. We got into a birthing room and, knowing my role as 'protector', I set to work trying to relax her down again – I dimmed all the lights, put on the music we had chosen, got her into some comfy clothing and helped her relax on to the bean bag in the corner of the room. Within half an hour everything was calm again and contractions were once again coming regularly. Our baby was born just an hour later!' – **James**

case study

The people around her
You also need to consider the people who will be in the room. For a straightforward birth it will be both of you and a midwife. That will be the minimum, but depending on your circumstances there may be more.

Do you need to protect you partner from the midwife? Absolutely! Not because the midwife is bad or dangerous – your partner just needs to feel comfortable with her midwife. In the majority of births, the midwife who will be caring for Mum during labour will be someone neither of you have met before, and so your role is even more important because you are someone she knows and trusts. To keep adrenalin levels down, your partner needs to feel surrounded by people she can trust and feels relaxed with.

Your role as protector does not stop there, though. You also need to protect your partner against *yourself*! During labour, your partner's senses will be heightened. Mother Nature gave this as a gift to labouring women so that they can sense any dangers around them, so that they can protect themselves (very important if you think about mammals giving birth in the wilderness where a passing bear could be a real possibility!). These heightened senses mean that during labour, your partner will sense any worries or tension coming from you. In a nutshell: *she will smell your fear!* If she senses that you are afraid or worried, it will trigger her fear and thus her adrenalin. This is why *you* preparing for *your* role during labour is so important. By being better prepared and informed, you will be calmer and more confident during labour and birth, and this will lead to less adrenalin for your partner and an easier birth. So, guys, if you skipped over my chapter in the previous section on what you are afraid of (see page 33), I would like you to go back and read it, please, as you now know why it is so important.

Your role is to focus on your partner and keep reassuring her. Overall, trust in *both* of your abilities and instincts, but be reassured that simply by reading this you will be better prepared. There may be points during the birth where you almost want to intervene, perhaps suggest that she uses some pain relief, for example. However, you have to remember that you can be a hindrance to the birthing process and your job is not to direct, but to protect. This can be easier said than done for many men due to our inbuilt 'fix-it' reflex (see box below). However, understanding that you have this impulse is the first step towards taking control of it.

The 'fix-it' reflex

Throughout this book you will find me referring to something called the male 'fix-it' reflex. Don't bother googling it, it isn't a medical term or even, as far as I am aware, a term used by anyone else. It's the phrase I use to explain the way men approach problems, which can have a real impact on labour and birth.

So what do I mean by the male 'fix-it' reflex?

As men we all have a subconscious instinctive behaviour pattern, which leads us to try to fix things or situations. After a few hundred arguments between myself and my wife after the birth of our first child, we finally realised what was going on (although I still fall foul of this one even now, despite being aware of it!). Steph would tell me about something she felt upset or anxious about and I would try to come up with suggestions for dealing with it. Rather than this helping, it only seemed to make her angry. You may well have experienced this yourself.

When it comes to emotional stuff, here is a key difference between men and women. While men look for practical solutions, women often just want to talk things through. They find it helpful to get things off their chest and feel listened to and supported. As Steph says 'Sometimes we just want to have a moan!'

Guys, with birth and the early days of parenthood, you need to worry less about fixing things. You need to rein in that urge and just try to be there for your partner. In summary: listen to her, reassure her and just be there for her.

When it comes to birth, reining in this 'fix-it' reflex is actually really important, although sometimes it is the most difficult time to do this, as it is likely to be the one occasion when we feel the reflex at its strongest. Some of the things women do and say in labour, the sounds they make or what they look like is a little scary – it can appear that they are in distress. We might have never heard them make those noises before (for example, she might moo like a cow), or say those things (such as swearing at you or the midwife). Our natural instinct tells us to intervene and get her help. We may do this in a number of ways, such as taking her to the hospital too early (because *we* want her there rather than *her* wanting to be there!), asking her if she wants pain relief or encouraging other forms of intervention. As we become fearful and anxious at her behaviour, she also begins to pick up on our emotional state, which then stimulates a release of adrenalin in her body, with all the negative consequences that can bring.

Dads, *it is not up to you* to make these decisions. You have to control your instinct to fix the situation. You have your roles and you should concentrate on those. If your partner does need help, she will ask for it, and you will have the 'code-word technique'. This is a technique I will explain fully on page 82 that you can both use when you want to communicate effectively with one another when, and if, things get tricky. This gives you total trust in the fact that if your partner wants you to do something for her, she has a way of asking for it that cannot be misinterpreted by you.

It is important to not try to fix things and interfere, as the moment you suggest some pain relief because *you* want to fix things, you have just become one of those grizzlies. You have suddenly suggested to her that she is not coping. Even if she is coping, she may suddenly feel that you are doubting her ability to cope. This breaks that protection and trust you are meant to be providing for her. If she doubts herself and becomes anxious, here comes that adrenalin.

It is an admirable quality to want to protect your partner and family. What you need to be aware of is that at certain points in life, and giving birth is one of them, your fix-it reflex can cause more harm than good. One of the ways you can learn to control this reflex is by being mindful of your role and what techniques you will be using as a birth partner. Keep preparing for the birth and allow yourselves to enjoy the experience, as it is a truly wonderful time – when you see what your partner is capable of doing and when you meet your child for the first time.

However, don't put your feet up yet … being your partner's protector is only half of your role …

Role two: be her advocate

What do I mean by 'be her advocate'? Put simply, to be an 'advocate' is to make sure your partner's wishes are heard and understood by other people. So, common sense should tell you that you cannot advocate successfully if you don't know what your partner's wishes are. Advocacy starts now – not just during labour! (I will focus on labour and birth here, but the same rules apply during pregnancy and when Baby joins you.)

In all things relating to labour and birth, you need to sit down together and talk things through. Look at what choices you might be presented with. Do keep reading because I discuss which key choices you need to consider in advance to fulfil this role in chapter 8. The aim is to talk things through and reach decisions that you both feel comfortable with. By simply doing this, you will become clearer on your role for the big day itself. I suggest you write a birth plan detailing these preferences, as you can give a copy to your midwife during labour, so that she knows in advance what kind of birth you would like her to help facilitate. It is also for your own benefit; having a copy you can refer to in the heat of the moment can be helpful. Again, there is more information about how to write this plan in chapter 8.

You should both be happy with your decisions, but if you cannot agree, then (sorry, guys) your partner's wishes come first. You have to accept this; a true advocate always puts forward the viewpoint of the person they are advocating for, regardless of their own feelings on the matter. It is also crucial for the birth process that your partner has complete trust that you will honour her wishes (as 'trust' means feeling safe, which means lots of oxytocin). So again, preparation here is the key to successfully advocating on behalf of your partner – you can only stick up for her if you know what she wants. When she is in labour, she may not be able to tell you. So how do you do it? Firstly, you can use your advocate role in conjunction with your protector role.

Most women when labouring in a good, sympathetic environment will 'zone out'. During contractions they will almost 'go into' themselves and be focused on what they are doing. You need to protect that state. *Nobody*, not you, not the midwife, no one should ask her a question during a contraction. If anyone does ask her a question, you will advocate for her, *not* by speaking on her behalf, but by gently asking the person to wait a moment and re-ask the question when the contraction has passed.

During labour, your partner may be offered pain relief or other interventions. Here, your role as her advocate is to ensure that the wishes that you have *discussed* are respected. Your partner will be vulnerable during labour; she will not generally feel in a position to debate or discuss – this will be *your* job. You may need to explain her preferences, you need to ensure that these are respected and that she isn't pressured into anything *she* isn't comfortable with. For any treatment, it will be Mum who will ultimately need to consent or not consent, but you can certainly back her up and reaffirm her wishes at each step, which takes a lot of the burden off her shoulders.

One question I get asked a lot is 'What if she changes her mind about something on the birth plan when she is actually in labour?' There is a special DaddyNatal technique for this … may I introduce 'code word'!

Code word – because you are *not* a mind reader

Firstly, all women are different during labour: some vocalise, some go into themselves and are almost silent, while with others the change is minimal. Your partner needs to follow her instincts and do whatever feels right for her, to allow her labour to progress. A very vocal, or conversely, completely silent partner can be very unsettling for the birth partner, but remember, it is *not* your job to try to second-guess how she is feeling – keep that 'fix-it' reflex under control!

The whole point about being empowered during birth is to do what feels right, and sometimes you don't know what that is until you are there in the moment. So there is no weakness in your partner changing her mind about something – this allows her to keep her options open. However, sometimes women in labour will say things that they do not really mean as part of an emotional release (which makes sense – her entire body and mind are undergoing a release as they release their baby). My wife, Steph, is a classic example of this! But she is not alone. I have lost count of the number of times I have heard this discussion played back to me:

Woman: 'Why did you let me have that? You knew I didn't want it!'

Partner: 'You asked for it!'

Woman: 'That's not the point. We talked about it and you knew I didn't want it!'

Partner: 'How was I to know? I'm not telepathic. I thought I was doing the right thing!'

Sometimes a woman in labour will change her mind about what she wants, but sometimes she will say all kind of things just as part of her release. What you both need is a safe way for her to change her mind about preferences, and a way for you to be *certain* that she really has changed her mind. Things can change during labour and you need a way for you to confirm those changes, without there being repercussions afterwards. So guys, listen up, here is your essential technique – a code word.

Yes, simple as it seems, a code word is an incredibly beneficial tool. As part of your birth preference discussions, you should sit down together and choose a code word that means something to you both. This should be a word or phrase that is easily remembered, but not one that you would be likely to use in everyday life. For example 'I want a lemon' would be very effective if Mum never, ever (in a million years) asks for a lemon, as the message couldn't be clearer!

Knowing that you are armed with a code word allows your partner to feel secure in the knowledge that if she needs to, she can signal to you she is very serious about something.

Once you have decided on your code word, this is how you will use it during labour.

1. If your partner asks for something that she stated she didn't want in your birth preferences, the first time you will ignore her.

2. If she asks a second time, simply ask her if she is sure, and if she says yes, confirm her choice by asking for the code word. If she gives you the code word, give her, or advocate for, what she wants.

Why do you follow these steps? Simply, by ignoring it the first time you are giving space for her to just be vocalising. Then by asking 'if she is sure' the second time she asks for the same thing, you are giving her just a moment to think about it, to question herself. If she says yes, by asking for your code word, you are empowering her to confirm her decision.

You do not need to go past these steps and keep on questioning her. If the code word is given *you do not* need to ask her again whether she is sure!

It is important to make sure this questioning is done sensitively – you are not doing this to tease or withhold, you are using it as a way of making sure you are truly advocating for what she wants at that moment.

This very simple technique, used correctly, can increase the trust you have in each other and it further enhances the positive birthing environment.

Please remember, though, that your role as an advocate does not end with the birth of your child, because once your child is born you will be advocating on your partner's wishes regarding the third stage of labour. If your partner has decided to have unassisted third stage (see page 68), one of you needs to let the midwife know. If you see an injection being prepared without having been asked whether it is wanted (rare, but I have known cases where this did happen) you may need to physically get in the way of the injection. This sounds like drastic action, but it's better to physically block an unwanted injection if it's being given without consent than Mum being injected with something she resolutely doesn't want or even knows she might have an adverse reaction to – until that conversation can be had.

You will have some decisions to make after the baby is born, including cord cutting, injections, examinations, feeding and skin-to-skin contact. All of these options are described in more detail in chapter 8. You should also be aware of these choices, discuss them beforehand and then ensure that those decisions made on behalf of your partner *and* your baby are respected.

'Amit was absolutely amazing. He was positive and kept doing the breathing with me. He held me, rocked me and understood what I was going through. He was the most supportive birth partner I could have imagined and I really feel we did it together. We have come out of it so much stronger too. I know the DaddyNatal techniques really helped him as he was just so confident.' – **Reshma**

case study

Your role during a Caesarean section

As a birth partner, your role during a Caesarean birth is just as important as during any other kind of birth – you are still there as your partner's protector and advocate.

In terms of being her protector, you are there to keep your partner as calm and reassured as possible. It would not be unusual if she felt anxiety (you may both be feeling anxious, even if it was a planned Caesarean), and your support, to be at her side, to keep talking to her and reassuring her throughout, is crucial. Remember that stress hormones cross the placenta, so by keeping Mum as calm as possible you are also helping your baby keep calm as he arrives into the world!

In your role as advocate, you are also there to ensure any wishes you have expressed on the birth plan have been understood. I cover this in more detail in the next chapter. Even if you had not planned for a Caesarean birth, there will still be birth preferences that may be able to be accommodated, such as finding out the sex of baby yourself, having skin-to-skin time after the birth and having your birth music playing in the background.

As Mum recovers from her Caesarean, your role as her protector and advocate continues, supporting her wishes to get appropriate painkillers as she needs, and continuing to be there offering her support and reassurance. Mum may find it difficult to move around or pick up your baby, so very practical and hands-on support is really crucial at this time.

Can I really be her birth partner?

If you are having concerns about being your partner's birth partner, listen up. Your partner wants you to be there. Your baby needs you to be there. So if you want to be at the birth, put in some effort and be the best birth partner you can be. You have the potential to truly affect the whole experience and outcome. By fulfilling the two key roles of being her protector and advocate your presence can increase the chances of you all having a positive birth experience.

Yes, this is an awesome responsibility and it can feel intimidating, but being prepared is the key. *Talk* about the choices and possibilities beforehand. It is very difficult to advocate for someone when you do not know what their preferences are.

You may come to the conclusion that you don't feel you can fulfil the roles of advocate and birth partner – and that is okay. You mustn't feel pressurised into it as then there is the risk of you having a detrimental effect on the birth, and you also deserve to be able to enjoy the experience too. In those circumstances, perhaps there is another family member or friend who your partner feels would be a good additional support. You could also think about hiring a doula. Doulas are professionally trained to provide support for expectant parents at the birth of their baby. They can support you both together through the birth, or a doula can even be a sole birth partner, if you feel very uncomfortable being there. You can find out more about the support doulas provide and see a list of those in your local area by visiting www.doula.org.uk. Ultimately, it is normal to feel nervous about the labour and birth, but it is about finding what is right for you as a couple.

CHAPTER 8

Birth preferences

You may have heard people talking about creating a 'birth plan', where you plan out how you and your partner would like the birth to go. However, I find the term 'birth plan' misleading. It isn't a plan of exactly how your birth will go; writing one with that concept in mind can lead to disappointment, guilt and perhaps even to birth trauma. All births are different, choices made may need to change, depending on how things progress, how your partner is feeling and other circumstances beyond your control. However, this does not mean that it is therefore better not to have thought about it – thinking about your preferences in advance is very helpful, especially when you find yourself faced with difficult decisions on the day. Instead I prefer to think of this document as a list of birth 'preferences'. Used in the right way, the list is an incredibly useful tool, especially for you, the birth partner, in your role as advocate (see the previous chapter, page 80).

Why should you have a birth plan?

Birth preferences, should be written *by both of you*. I would suggest starting to research this and your options around weeks 30–32 of the pregnancy. By simply writing your birth preferences, it will encourage you both to look at the options available and give you an opportunity to research and discuss them.

Guys, if when writing out these birth preferences, your preference is not the same as that of your partner, at some point you must wholeheartedly accept *her* preference. It is important that she can have faith in you to protect her wishes as well as her environment; that is your role.

Once you have both researched and are happy with your preferences, write them out clearly, concisely and in a logical order. You do not need to write the reasons for your preferences, just list them logically. If you can, keep your plan to a single side of A4. Make sure you have a few copies packed in the hospital bags (see page 115). When you get to hospital, give one copy to your midwife and keep another to hand for you to refer to, if you need to.

I will give you a little more detail on some of the choices you may wish to consider. However, this doesn't mean that this book should be your sole source of research to make an informed choice. Read around, gain different insights into your possible choices and find preferences that feel right for you.

Key choices one: where do you want to give birth?

This is often a decision that can change as you progress through the pregnancy. This is fine; the initial decision you make does not have to be one you stick with.

Basically you have three main choices: home birth, a private birth centre or a hospital birth.

Home birth

A home birth is exactly that – giving birth to your baby in your own home. Midwives will attend you during the birth. They will bring a home birth kit, which has all the equipment they may use. Mum still has the options of using gas and air or pethidine during the labour (see pages 100–7 for more on pain-relief options), and in the event of any concerns about Mum or Baby the decision can be made to transfer to hospital.

Experience has shown me that, especially for first-time parents, it is commonly Dad who will have reservations about having a home birth. Statistically, home births are as safe as hospital births and have better birth outcomes. The main reason women in labour will be transferred into hospital is due to a request for additional pain relief rather than a medical necessity. In the event of medical support being needed, it is rare that during birth things go from being fine to urgent quickly. More often than not there are warning signs – and that is why you have a midwife with you – to look for those signs and if she is at all concerned she will organise a transfer.

If you have opted for a home birth and for whatever reason, even during labour, you change your mind, you can.

One of the benefits of a home birth is that it is an environment that you are both comfortable in, so in terms of your protector role, there are fewer potential 'grizzlies' (see page 74) to keep at bay, and that is certainly easier. But it is crucial that you are both really happy and comfortable with the decision to have a home birth, because if it doesn't feel the right place to give birth for *both* of you, then the chances are adrenalin will kick in, which makes the whole thing counterproductive anyway.

Private birth centre

If you can afford one of these, they are just as they sound (they are 'private' so are not open to everyone and are exclusively dedicated to birthing). The environment tends to be less medicalised and more conducive to birth than a typical hospital delivery room, and you will have more freedom with regard to the services provided (for example, there would be an increased likelihood of being able to have a water birth). Many also have the facilities for Dad to stay once Baby is born, although this is starting to happen in some NHS hospitals as well.

Hospital

When opting to birth in a hospital environment your first choice will be which hospital, as there may be two or three within your area to choose from. In making your decision, you can see if the hospital offer tours (which will help you get a feel for the place), see what experiences friends and family may have had, but also, crucially, it is helpful to look at the statistics for your chosen hospital. What are their rates for assisted birth and Caesarean section? If you want to increase the likelihood of having a natural birth, then choosing a hospital where this is more likely to be achieved statistically might be something you wish to consider. A great website which enables you to compare hospitals' maternity statistics is www.birthchoiceuk.com.

Even if you have chosen to have a hospital birth, your choices do not necessarily end there. There will often still be a few choices to make, as many hospitals now divide their birthing facilities into a delivery suite and a midwife-led unit.

Midwife-led units are usually located adjacent to the delivery suite, but often they offer rooms that are less medicalised than full birthing suites, and they often contain choices such as water birth, and fewer beds and more active birthing facilities such as bean bags, birth stools, birth couches and so forth. Usually to use a midwife-led facility you need to be considered a 'low-risk' pregnancy. If Mum has been under the care of a consultant for the pregnancy, but would like to use the facilities of a midwife-led unit, speak to your doctor about it, as depending on the reason for your consultant-led care, they may write on your notes that they support you having midwife-led care for birth.

Otherwise, a delivery suite will usually lead you into a traditional birth room, where your role of protector of the environment comes to the fore! You can still use birth balls and similar equipment in these rooms. If you are in one of these rooms for monitoring or to be on a drip, for example, remember that this does not prevent Mum sitting on a yoga ball or using positions such as all-fours or kneeling. Just because there is a bed in the room this does not mean that she needs to lie on it, and if she has the energy, encouraging her into positions where she can harness gravity will be very beneficial to progressing labour more quickly.

Key choices two: is there anything in particular you want to have/use at the birth?

Wherever you plan to have your baby, a key birth preference is to have thought about the practical, tangible things that you *can* plan. While you might not be able to control certain things that present themselves, there are a lot of things that you can control. For the midwives who will be at your birth, it is helpful for them to know what kind of environment or techniques you are aiming to use.

If you and your partner have been learning particular movements or positions you want to use for the birth, or particular breathing techniques, also put these on your birth plan. This helps the midwife to encourage you both with your techniques, as otherwise she won't know you have these skills to hand!

Whether you want a dimmed room, music playing, people to speak in low voices, to use a scent to aid relaxation – these are all things you can control about the labour, and if you are proactive, they are also things you can take control of from the start. Sorting these things out is very much the birth partner's domain, too, as Mum is going to be a little busy dealing with her contractions. So, when you are writing your birth plan, spend less time worrying about things that you cannot control (such as needing an assisted delivery, for example) and more time focused on the proactive things you know you can do, which in turn will aid the chances of you both having the birth you want.

Some things you write down may be preferences that are not guaranteed – such as birthing in a birth pool – but it is important they are on there too. Yes, it can be disappointing if not every preference you wish for can be realised, but there are many ways of having a positive birth. Having every single birth preference fulfilled is not the only way to have an amazing birth experience. Sometimes the path changes, but it doesn't make the journey any less fantastic. However, you can only have the option of having something if you are first prepared to ask for it.

Birth pools

Wherever you decide to give birth, you may want to consider using a birth pool. You can hire one of these to use at home, or many hospitals and birth centres have access to one. Water is, in itself, a great pain relief, so it is definitely an option worth exploring, as are different types of rooms that may be available in your own particular hospital – all hospitals are different.

Key choices three: how do you feel about induction?

Induction of labour basically means kick-starting labour rather than letting it start of its own accord. (There are a variety of methods for doing this, see pages 98–100 for more on this.) Induction may be offered for a medical reason, when medical professionals believe it is safer for Mum and Baby to have the birth earlier. However, it can also be offered if labour has not started by itself by around 10 days after the due date.

Why does this all matter? It matters because induction is a common intervention, and, as with any intervention, there are risks associated with it that you should be aware of.

Choosing whether or not to be induced is often not an easy decision because there will be risks to consider on both sides. If you are being offered induction for a medical reason (such as pre-eclampsia, see page 57) the medical professionals should explain to you both the risks of induction, but also the risks of continuing the pregnancy.

If you are being offered induction because your partner is now 41 weeks pregnant, then again you should have the risks of induction explained to you, as well as the risks attached to prolonging a pregnancy past 42 weeks.

Ultimately, if you end up in this position, you need to make sure you are being given all the information on both sides, so that you can balance the risks when making a decision on whether to be induced or not. As with many things in life, there is not a simple 'right' or 'wrong' answer; it becomes about working out what risks you are prepared to take, understanding the measures you can use to minimise those risks and doing what you feel is right in *your* circumstances.

If you proceed with induction, that is your choice. However, it will be classed on your medical notes that you consented to induction – so if you are going to consent to something that affects both Mum and Baby, just make sure you are informed about the decision you are making. Induction is *always* a choice. Sometimes it is a choice that seems obvious (especially when this is for urgent medical reasons), but if it is being offered because there is a belief that Baby may be 'big' or because Baby is approaching 42 weeks even though everything looks healthy in the antenatal checks, then it is a little less clear-cut. You should never feel that you 'have to be' induced because your baby has not arrived by 10 days after the due date.

Chapter 11 will go into this in more detail and I will give you a technique to use to help you weigh up the issues involved. It is important that you make an informed choice on this one, as statistics show that, depending on your hospital, up to 32 per cent of labours are now induced, and it is accepted (and even stated in National Institute for Health and Clinical Excellence/NICE guidance) that there is an increased likelihood of requiring pain relief and an assisted delivery with induction. If this is something you do not want, you owe it to yourselves to at least consider all the options thoroughly first.

In first-time parents, there is also evidence suggesting that induction leads to an increased likelihood of Caesarean section. One study[1] found an increased Caesarean section rate of 20 per cent for women being induced with their first baby. This study concluded that induction had a strong correlation with Caesarean birth in first-time mums, and thus a decrease in induction may lead to a decrease in the number of Caesarean births for first-time mums. In fact, another study[2] found induction increased the chance of a Caesarean section by three times for first-time mothers. These risks are becoming more understood and it appears that there are an increasing percentage of parents, not least among those we teach, who are carefully weighing up their options when it comes to induction.

So the obvious question is ...

Induction – What are the options?

OPTION ONE: Go natural!

The least invasive way of inducing is by using natural methods to kick-start things. Whether these are old wives' tales or there is something more to them is up for debate, but many parents feel that they are worth a try as that due date approaches and passes! Some of the key ones you might want to try are:

- **Sex.** Women are not always in the mood when they are very heavily pregnant, but making love releases oxytocin, which is responsible for labour beginning and progressing. Semen also contains prostaglandins, which help soften the cervix.
- **Eat some spicy food.** Some swear by this; others say it has no effect ... but worth a try if you like spicy food!
- **Nipple stimulation.** Again this can stimulate the release of the hormone oxytocin. Mum can try some gentle nipple stimulation in the shower or if you are having sex, include this as part of that.
- **Fresh pineapple.** Eaten fresh, this is believed to increase the production of prostaglandins. However, for this to be effective it is believed that large amounts need to be eaten. So, again, it may be worth a try if your other half enjoys pineapple, but perhaps not if she doesn't like them!
- **Walking.** This may allow gravity to encourage the baby to drop further into the pelvis, stimulating the release of oxytocin. Taking a walk together is a great idea. Just make sure that she isn't too tired out as she will need some energy should labour begin!
- **Acupressure or acupuncture.** Many testify to this getting labour going, and it is usually a nice relaxing way of achieving it too!

However, with all of these options, please bear in mind that you are still attempting an induction, even though these are gentle and natural ways. This just means that some of these methods may come with their own side effects, such as an upset tummy from the spicy food, or labour coming on very quickly from an acupressure treatment.

OPTION TWO: Ask to be monitored
If you would prefer not to be induced, then that is your choice. The National Institute for Health and Clinical Excellence

(NICE) guidelines state 'If a woman chooses not to have induction of labour, her decision should be respected. Healthcare professionals should discuss the woman's care with her from then on.' If you decline the induction of labour, from 42 weeks you should be offered regular monitoring to check how your baby is getting on, and if there are any concerns at all professionals can let you know so that you can reassess your decision to wait.

OPTION THREE: Medical induction

If you choose to go ahead with a medical induction, there are several possible methods that can be used. This will usually be determined following monitoring and a vaginal examination to assess what is known as Mum's 'Bishop's score'. This check is to see how 'favourable' her cervix is – for example, whether her body has already started making progress in terms of preparation for labour. If her cervix is deemed 'favourable' it means that induction is more likely to be successful. However, if the check shows that the cervix is 'unfavourable' (i.e. the body has not yet started preparing itself for labour) then induction is less likely to work – which all makes sense when you think about it!

Methods of medical induction

The methods of induction, depending on the assessment of the Bishop's score, are:

- **A 'sweep'.** A sweep is normally carried out by a midwife. Similar to a vaginal examination, the midwife will insert her fingers into your partner's vagina, stretching the cervix and sweeping her fingers across the membrane. Sometimes this can stimulate contractions within the next day or so. It doesn't always work and often they will try two or three times before looking at other forms of induction.

Risks include: accidentally breaking the waters during the examination, and as with any vaginal examination, there is always a risk of the introduction of infection.

■ **Pessary, tablet or gel.** This contains prostaglandin, a hormone that helps to soften the cervix, and is inserted into the vagina.

Risks include: uterine hyperstimulation, which means contractions last longer and come more frequently than should be safely expected. Uterine hyperstimulation can lead to uterine rupture, foetal distress and other associated complications.

■ **Artificial rupture of the membranes.** This simply means artificially breaking the bag of waters around Baby. The midwife uses an instrument, not dissimilar to a crochet hook, which she inserts through the cervix to rupture it. Mum does not feel any pain, although, like a vaginal examination, it may be uncomfortable. The aim is to remove the cushion of water between Baby and the cervix, to put more pressure on the cervix, to increase the pace of labour. One review of the studies considering the impact of artificial rupture of the membranes reported that the evidence did not show that it made the first stage of labour go any quicker, and that there was a possible link to an increase in Caesarean section. They concluded that rupturing the membranes should not be routinely used to speed up labours.[3]

Risks include: increase in the intensity of contractions felt by Mum, foetal distress.

■ **Syntocinon.** This is an artificial form of oxytocin, the hormone needed for labour. It is normally administered through an intravenous (IV) drip in the hand. Syntocinon stimulates contractions, which can be very strong. Guidance under the National Institute for Clinical Excellence (NICE) states that anyone being offered syntocinon should be advised that because of the nature of the intervention the likelihood of needing increased pain relief is also increased.

Risks include: uterine hyperstimulation and therefore the associated risks including uterine rupture and foetal distress, as well as possible side effects, such as nausea, headaches, fall in blood pressure and heart problems.

Remember, this is just an overview to get you started. Research your options, make sure you get balanced information and follow your instincts.

Good resources to use for more information include:

Birth Rights – An organisation that provides legal information and advice on the law relating to women and birth – www. birthrights.org.uk.

Birth Choice UK – Covers options around place of birth as well as evidence-based resources on various aspects of birth – www.birthchoiceuk.com.

Key choices four: what forms of pain relief do you want to use?

You might assume that labour is always painful. However, pain is actually quite a debated term in respect of labour and birth. Bear in mind that childbirth as portrayed on TV shows and films as being agonising and dramatic is not always representative of the reality.

Childbirth is not always painful and the type of antenatal preparation that your partner decides on will make a massive difference to her experience. My wife, Steph, who is also an antenatal educator, likens it to preparation for a marathon. If you were going to put your body through an intense, and possibly long, physical endurance event, wouldn't you prepare your body for it? Would you prepare your mind for it? If you didn't, then surely the experience would be much more diffi-cult and, yes, more painful than if you didn't?

The reality is that women experience labour in different ways. Through our own practice with thousands of parents we have worked with many who have not described it as 'painful' but rather as 'powerful' or 'intense'. Many have described con-tractions as feelings of 'tightening' or 'pressure', so there are many words that can also be used that are more descriptive than painful.

Please note, I am *not* saying that women are lying about labour pain! Some women will have been through very pain-ful labours – all I am saying here is that different women feel different things. Much of this depends on the kind of prepara-tion you both do in advance of the birth, the environment you create and the choices you make on the day.

The irony here is that if you go into birth believing that it is going to be horrendously painful, then the likelihood is that this is exactly what will happen, as it becomes a self-fulfilling prophecy. Think about what you learnt about earlier in terms of fear and adrenalin, and the effects this will have on slowing or stalling labour, therefore making it more difficult. If women go into the birth believing it is going to be horribly painful, they will be scared, and if they are scared they produce adren-alin … and then they have the long, drawn-out and painful labour they believed they would!

So, the key choices when it comes to pain relief are:

OPTION ONE: Natural techniques for minimising or preventing pain

■ **Specialist antenatal classes.** As discussed above, labour does not necessarily mean unbearable pain. The sensations Mum will experience depend a lot on her birthing environ-ment, her birthing companions and her labour preparations.

There are now numerous antenatal classes that mums can take to learn techniques for a more comfortable labour and birth.

Research classes such as HypnoBirthing or Natal Hypnotherapy. While these are often not the 'cheap alternative', they do have fantastic results. Be prepared to practise what you learn, which often includes breathing techniques, relaxation exercises, massage and so forth. Check out the resources section on page 221 for more information on birth classes.

- **Using water.** Using warm water during labour can relax Mum and make her contractions more bearable – just as you might have a bath to help with a back or stomach ache. In fact, a review found that women who used water for labour felt less pain, were less likely to use drugs or have an epidural.

Remember, if Mum would like to try to use water, she does not have to give birth in it as well. It is fine to use the pool and then get out in time for the actual birth. Equally, if Mum is in the pool and is very comfortable, so that she doesn't want to get out, that is a choice too! Your baby will not try to breathe until she is in air, so a baby born under water will continue to receive oxygen via the umbilical cord until she is brought up to the surface.

OPTION TWO: Medicalised forms of pain relief

- **TENS** (transcutaneous electrical nerve stimulation). A maternity TENS machine is a hand-held controller attached to sticky pads placed on Mum's back. The machine emits pulses of electrical energy that may stimulate the body to release endorphins, the body's natural painkillers.

Advantages of TENS

- Mum can continue to remain mobile.
- Mum can control the TENS machine herself and use it for as long as she wants.
- TENS machines are completely safe for both Mum and Baby and there are no lasting side effects.
- She can use it by herself — without a medical professional being present, though someone will need to help her position the pads on her back.
- You can use TENS machines at a home birth.
- TENS are easy to use, but you both need to read the instructions beforehand — perhaps well before you actually need to use it!

Disadvantages of TENS

- Mum will need someone to help position the pads on her back.
- The TENS machine may only help with pain relief during early labour.
- It costs between £20 and £30 to hire — so this may be an expense you don't want.
- The TENS machine may need to be taken off if Baby's heart has to be monitored electronically.
- If Mum wants to use a birthing pool or bath, she cannot use the TENS machine in water.
- If Mum wants her back massaged, this will be more difficult — because the pads will be in the way.

■ **Entonox.** Also known as 'gas and air', this is a colourless, odourless gas, which is composed of half oxygen and half nitrous oxide. If Mum inhales it at the onset of a contraction it can provide a calming effect and soothe pain.

Gas and air can be used wherever you give birth. If you are having a home birth the midwife can bring it with her.

Advantages of entonox

- Entonox is fast-acting and is very easy to use, though you may need a bit of coaching from your midwife to get the timing right.
- Mum can control how and when she uses entonox and if she doesn't like it or it doesn't suit her for some reason, she can stop.
- Entonox doesn't remain in Mum's body. As soon as she stops breathing it in, the gas and air is cleared by her lungs and any side effects will cease.
- Entonox takes the edge off the pain of contractions.
- It's safe for baby and the extra oxygen that Mum breathes in may even be good for her and her baby.
- The baby doesn't require extra monitoring while Mum is using it.
- Mum can still use entonox if she is labouring in water or in a birth pool.

Disadvantages of entonox

- Entonox is only a mild painkiller.
- Mum may start to feel drowsy, light-headed or nauseous and she could be sick.
- Mum may experience tingling, a pins-and-needles sensation or temporary muscle cramps or spasms in her wrist or ankle joints.

- **Pethidine.** Part of the opiate drug family, this painkiller also has properties to aid relaxation. It should be available wherever you give birth, including at home.

Advantages of pethidine
- Pethidine can be given by a midwife, so Mum does not need a doctor to see her first.
- Pethidine can help Mum to relax and get some rest.
- Pethidine may help Mum to avoid having an epidural if she is finding her contractions hard to cope with.
- It can be used at a home birth.

Disadvantages of pethidine
- Pethidine provides only limited relief from labour pain.
- One in three women find opiate drugs such as pethidine unpleasant, and the side effects may make it more difficult for them to cope with labour.
- It can make women feel sick or vomit, even if they take an anti-sickness drug.
- Pethidine may make women feel dizzy, elated or depressed.
- It crosses the placenta and may affect the baby's breathing, causing them to be drowsy for several days.
- It may be more difficult to get breastfeeding started. This is because pethidine has crossed the placenta to Baby and may affect her rooting and sucking reflexes.
- Pethidine takes 30 minutes to work, so Mum will still need other coping methods while the drug begins to take effect.

■ **Epidural.** During an epidural, painkilling drugs are passed into the small of the woman's back via a fine tube by an anaesthetist. It is a regional anaesthetic, so the drug works on the local nerves to numb the region around Mum's abdomen.

Advantages of an epidural
- Effective form of pain relief during labour.
- Mum will feel less pain, and perhaps even no pain.
- If Mum has high blood pressure, it can help to lower it. So in some cases, this can increase her chances of having a vaginal birth.
- It can be topped up with stronger local anaesthetic if Mum needs an unplanned Caesarean.

Disadvantages of an epidural
- For about one in eight women the epidural doesn't work well enough and only numbs parts of the tummy rather than the whole abdomen and sometimes the legs.
- Though epidurals work fairly quickly, Mum may have to wait until an anaesthetist is available to administer it. It then takes about 20 minutes to set up the epidural, and around another 20 minutes to work once the anaesthetic has been injected. So setting up and giving it takes a lot longer than most other types of pain relief.
- It may make Mum feel shivery or she may develop a fever.
- Your partner will need to stay in bed, as her legs are likely to feel very weak or heavy. Even if she is able to shuffle around on the bed, she won't be able to walk around.
- It can affect your partner's ability to wee, so she may need a catheter until the epidural has worn off after the birth.

Disadvantages of an epidural continued

- Mum will need more monitoring to make sure her blood pressure is okay, and that Baby is okay too.
- Your partner is more likely to have labour assisted with a syntocinon drip (see page 99).
- The second stage of labour (the part where Mum gives birth) can last longer and Mum may not feel an urge to push, which may lead to even more intervention, such as a ventouse or forceps birth.
- There is more chance of your baby needing to be born with the aid of forceps or ventouse. This may be because epidurals, and the limit they put on what position Mum can get into, can make it difficult for your baby to move into the best position for birth or descend through the pelvis.
- There is a 1 per cent risk of Mum developing a severe headache. This can happen if the epidural needle punctures the bag of fluid that surrounds the spinal cord, causing a fluid leak.
- There is a very small risk of nerve damage, leaving Mum with a numb patch on her leg or foot, or a weak leg. The risk is about one in 1,000 for temporary nerve damage and one in 13,000 for permanent damage.

Key choices five: what about after the birth?

The moment your baby has arrived, there are still a plenty of choices open to you that you may want to have considered and include on your birth preferences. Things you may want to consider are:

- **Third stage of labour.** It is helpful to have your preferences about the third stage noted. This is basically about whether the placenta is birthed naturally or with medical assistance. Both choices have different benefits and risks for you to consider, so research them and then go with what you feel is right for you both. Remember, though, that it is just a preference you are expressing. Mum can always change her mind on the day if she wishes.
- **Cord-clamping**. Up until recently, it was fairly standard to clamp a baby's cord soon after birth. Guidance is now shifting and it is becoming more common practice, if Mum and Baby are well, to allow the cord to finish pulsating before clamping it. This allows the baby to get all of her blood volume from the placenta (where some of it will still be, even at birth). Find out if delayed cord-clamping is standard at your hospital. If it is something that you want, just make sure it is included on the birth plan.
- **Cutting the cord**. Once the cord is clamped, do you want to be the one to cut it? Some guys worry about this, but there is no need to. Only do it if you want to, and if you are not sure then keep the option open and see how you feel at the time. Neither Mum nor Baby can feel anything, so there is nothing to worry about there. You will be given some surgical scissors to use and when you do so, you'll need to be firm about it! The midwives will guide you through it and many dads enjoy doing this as part of their rite of passage to fatherhood!
- **Skin-to-skin.** When your baby is born, your immediate choice is where do you first put her? Newborn babies bond

via touching and smelling and this is one of the reasons why skin-to-skin contact is thought to be a such a great idea. It simply means placing your baby straight on to Mum's chest after birth. This immediate skin-to-skin contact also has massive benefits, including helping to regulate Baby's body temperature and heartbeat and increasing the likelihood of successful breastfeeding. If there is a reason why Mum can't (or doesn't want) to have skin-to-skin for some reason, then how about you? Dads can also bond with their baby in this way and, if you would like to, all you need to do is take off your top (perhaps wear a button-down shirt to make this easier) and cuddle your baby to keep her warm and calm, while she gets to know you and starts to take in the world around her.

- **Vitamin K.** This is one of the first medical choices that your newborn will be offered – the vitamin K injection helps her blood clot (since babies are born with very little vitamin K in their system). Your midwife should give you information about this during the pregnancy, so that you can make an informed decision in advance. Therefore make sure that you both sit down and look over this literature. There are alternatives, such as having the vitamin K administered orally over several doses rather than injected in one large dose. Again, do your research and make a decision that feels right for your family.

Key choices six: planning a Caesarean birth

If you are planning a Caesarean birth, you can absolutely still write a birth plan and express basic preferences for the birth – it is still the birth of your baby!

Your birth plan should be personal to you both and discussed in advance with the midwife caring for you on the day – so that everyone is aware of your preferences. Be mindful of this in your role as advocate, as Mum may be feeling preoccupied or anxious in the lead-up, and find it difficult to have these conversations herself.

The following list of suggestions is not exhaustive, merely here to give you some ideas of how many preferences you are still able to express when planning a Caesarean birth. These are some of the preferences you may want to consider:

- If a general anaesthetic is used for the Caesarean section, do you want to keep your baby naked (albeit wrapped up to keep warm!) so that Mum can see her as she was when she arrived into the world, rather than washed and bathed already?
- Would you like to have the curtain dropped for the moment of birth, so you can see baby arriving into the world?
- Would you like photographs to be taken of the birth?
- Would you like the theatre to be as quiet as possible (from talking) at the moment of birth?
- Would you like any music played during the birth?
- Would you like to discover the sex of your baby yourself or have it announced?
- Would you like your baby lifted out on to Mum for immediate skin-to-skin contact where possible?
- Who would you like to cut the cord?

If you have not been planning for a Caesarean birth, but those are the circumstances you find yourself in, it can be more difficult to have a plan ready. You may want to consider a couple of aspects that are really important to you regardless of the birth, so that you can remember to ask for them, such as skin-to-skin contact after the birth or how you find out the sex of the baby.

A final word on the birth preferences …

By writing your birth preferences out together, you will gain an understanding of how you both feel about the various choices. This is crucial for the birth partner, in your role as advocate, since it is through understanding these preferences that you can advocate from a position of knowledge. Only through fully understanding these preferences can you have complete faith in each other. As the birth partner, your role is to have those preferences respected during labour (if for some reason a preference cannot be followed, keep asking the advocate's favourite question 'why' until you are satisfied that you have all the information).

Communication in all things is so important – none more so than planning your birth preferences. Spending some time researching and writing your preferences together will help you better understand the process and each other. In all things parenting, you are a team and that starts *now*!

'The skills I learnt through Dean's classes really helped Carla and I through our birth. I was able the challenge the midwives (when necessary) and this was down to the knowledge I had gained. I truly believe that if it wasn't for this knowledge of our options and my role, we would have been induced immediately, as the midwife advised. It was only after challenging her that we were informed of all the options and how long we could safely wait before the risks increased.

Friday – We went into hospital the day before our due date, after Carla's waters broke. She was monitored and we came home, having been asked to come back the following day for further monitoring.

Saturday — On our due date we went back for monitoring. As contractions hadn't started, the midwife told us we would be booked in to be induced that night. I asked what our options were as it felt we were being told what was going to happen to us rather than asked and given options. The midwife went on to tell us in more detail what they could do. She gave us some time to think about it and we decided that we would leave the induction as long as we safely could. She booked us in for further monitoring the next morning, followed by an induction the following night.

That night Carla lay in the bath willing our baby to come on his own. We went to bed and contractions started at midnight. Carla described how she felt really calm, in control and relieved.

Sunday — We were monitored in the morning as planned and came home again. At home Carla kept mobile and positive. The contractions became a lot stronger and were regular for an hour, so we called the hospital. The midwife asked Carla not to come in until the contractions were "taking her breath away".

Carla had a bath and could feel her contractions become a lot stronger. She had a contraction that seemed to knock her, so I said to Carla "How about your polar bear position to slow things down a bit?" She went into the position, which seemed to give her a minute to regain her focus. It had been about an hour since ringing the hospital and we both felt it was time to go in.

The maternity ward seemed busy and Carla leant against me as we waited to be seen. When she was examined, the midwife said to Carla, "We need to get you into a delivery room, you're 7 cm, you've done so well." I was so proud of her.

The midwife settled us into a delivery room. Carla leant against the side of the bed and had the urge to bear down. She was checked again and was now 9 cm dilated. She used some gas and air and the midwife asked if she would like any more pain relief, but she said she didn't need any.

Three hours after arriving at hospital baby Alfie was born weighing 3.5 kg (8 lb) and labour was very calm and controlled. I felt very clear on my role and how I could support Carla to have the birth we both wanted.

Having learned the DaddyNatal techniques and information was a blessing to us. I learned so much and it prepared us for the most important thing we would ever do – bringing our Alfie into the world.

Why wouldn't you prepare yourself for such a huge life event?' – **Brian**

case study

CHAPTER 9

Tools of the trade – your labour kit

Time to get practical now – what will you need to fulfil your role as this fantastic birth partner that you are going to be?

Birth bags

An important part of your role as birth partner is looking after the 'birth bags', which are the bags containing all the things you'll need for the birth. These days you can even buy birth bags with 'all the essentials' for Mum or for Baby. However, as a good birth partner, you will go a little further than that.

First up, it's a good idea to have three bags: one for Mum, one for Baby and one for you. Now you might think that Mum will probably pack the bags for herself and the baby so you don't have to worry about those, right? *Wrong!*

Even if Mum has got those bags all prepared, you need to be involved; you need to know what is in each bag and also *where* it is in the bag. Trust me, dads, 'man-looking' during labour is not going to win you any brownie points. When Mum says she needs something from the bag, you saying you can't find it (or worse – having her have to break her concentration to come and find it for herself) will just not do. I've been there and it's not pretty!

Your bag

There are plenty of resources you can check out to find out what should be packed in Mum's bag and in Baby's bag, so in this book I am just going to detail what should go in Dad's bag. The bag itself doesn't have to be huge, but there are some very handy bits of kit to have ready:

Essential things to pack:

- **Flexible straw.** I consider this an absolute birth essential and one that often gets commented on by dads that have been through my classes. Keeping Mum hydrated is extremely important. Labour is all about the uterus contracting and the uterus itself is a muscle. Now any of you athletic types will know that muscles need to be hydrated to work effectively, so keeping fluid intake up is essential. Sips, little and often, is a good rule of thumb for this one.
- **When labour is very advanced,** you will find that your partner simply may not have the energy or inclination to hold a cup for herself and, honestly, trying to hold a cup to your partner's lips is only going to end one way: your partner wet and not happy with you. By simply taking a stock of flexible straws you can hold the cup near to your partner, allowing her to turn her head and take a sip whenever she wants to.
- **Lip balm.** Using deep-breathing techniques can be very dehydrating for Mum and can lead to dry lips and mouth. Should she use entonox (gas and air) during the labour, this is even more likely. Having a normal stick of lip balm Mum can apply during the labour can bring her great relief.
- **Flannel.** Pack a couple of new flannels. These can be placed under a warm tap and used as a warm compress on Mum's lower back during labour to offer relief from any discomfort there, or placed under a cold tap and used as a cold compress on Mum's face towards the end of first stage of labour

and/or in the second stage of labour. A cold flannel when Mum is working hard can offer amazing relief (giving birth can be a hot and sweaty job!) and revitalise her during that important time.

- **Small change.** Have lots of coins ready in your bag. You will need them for the parking meter, for vending machines and everything else you can possibly imagine. Trust me when I say you can never have too much change.
- Food and drink. Make sure you take a supply of food and drink for yourself. Glucose energy drinks are great – although you might want to avoid the ones with added caffeine or taurine. You should also make sure you have some food that you can leave in your bag until it is needed, such as cereal bars, nuts or crisps. Ideally, make some sandwiches when labour begins and pop them into your bag too. This is a job you should just do yourself. *Do not* ask your partner to prepare your sandwiches, rely on stopping en route to pick some up or start asking her where things are to make them. Just take care of this task quietly and quickly. You need to keep your energy up in order to be able to look after your partner and you will need sustenance to do this. You do not want to be passing out at a crucial moment in the birth because you have not eaten for hours, nor do you want to be the dad who misses the birth because he was in the café! When preparing your snacks, be aware of packing *anything* that is strong-smelling. As discussed in chapter 7 (see page 77), a labouring woman's senses are heightened during labour and strong smells may turn her stomach or cause a distraction.
- **Glucose tablets or lozenges.** Get some of these and make sure they are in your bag, but don't hog them. They are great for you, but they are also excellent for Mum if she needs some extra energy. Make sure they are just glucose and do not contain any additives such as caffeine.

- **Birth preferences.** Make sure you have at least a couple of copies of your birth preferences sheet in your bag: one for your own reference in your role as advocate and one for the midwife. Don't try to remember everything you have discussed together; it is okay to refer back to your birth preferences sheet if you need to. Refer back to chapter 8 for more on what should go on this list.
- **Music.** Music for labour should not just be chosen at random or because you like a particular song. Music is an important tool in creating a positive, safe environment that will help labour to progress naturally. Ideally, you will want to use music that Mum has practised relaxing to already (so that when she hears it, she instantly associates positive, relaxing feelings with it) or gentle music that has good memories attached to it, which will help the oxytocin flow. During the birth of our second baby (our daughter Willow), Steph and I played the Snow Patrol album *Eyes Open* – an album that we had listened to together a lot when we first met and had a lot of positive associations with.

CHAPTER 10

Labour: your step-by-step roadmap

Okay, you understand the basics of labour, you are clear on your role, you have some great techniques up your sleeve to use, you have your labour kit, your dad's birth bag and birth preferences at the ready … This chapter is going to help you build on all this even more and break down each part of labour for you, as it can be useful to have an understanding of what is likely to happen and when, what signs might suggest that things are moving along (especially as usually it's us men who feel the burden of making sure we get to the hospital in time!). Medically, labour is referred to as being made up of three stages (see page 65), but in reality you may find that you experience this differently.

The first stage: pre labour and active labour

You will know from reading chapter 6 on labour basics that during this first part of labour (see page 65) your partner's body is working hard to open the cervix. So what exactly should you be doing at this point?

- **Keep breathing.** Make sure that Mum is taking deep, slow breaths; the uterus is a muscle and it needs oxygen to work. Deep breathing will also help her to relax and keep calm – it is, after all, a well-known technique for overcoming phobias and calming down before public speaking!
- **Have a cuddle.** Try to ensure that you are both staying relaxed to aid the production of the birth hormone oxytocin (to get labour moving!) and prevent the production of any adrenalin through fear or worry. Keep reassuring her.
- **If it's night-time when things begin,** you should both try to get some sleep and rest. Forcing yourself to stay awake during the night causes the production of adrenalin and so is detrimental for Mum anyway. While it is true that your partner might not get the best night's sleep she has ever had, hopefully she will doze and rest a little, and keep those adrenalin levels down.
- **If it's daytime,** just try to be gently active. The best thing you can do during this time is to just continue with your lives or go for a walk. During this stage with our second baby, my wife insisted we went to the shops! Walking around or staying upright on a birthing ball will make use of gravity, since when Baby is pressing down on the cervix at the bottom of the uterus, this encourages it to open more quickly.
- **Stay where it is comfortable.** In all seriousness, though, Mum should be where she feels most comfortable. If you think back to what I discussed about your role during labour and protecting the environment (see pages 74–76), the best place to labour early on is in your own comfortable surroundings. Keeping oxytocin levels high and adrenalin levels low is also important for keeping labour moving along, and using relaxation techniques and helping keep Mum positive and calm is really important for this too.
- **Think food.** Dad, you also need to make sure, if labour has started during the day, that Mum is keeping her energy

levels up, so make sure she is eating and drinking. Again, you do not want her to dehydrate, as this will make it harder for the uterine muscle to work and can cause pain. She might not be particularly in the mood to eat, so make small, tempting snacks and try to keep feeding her.

■ **Bathroom breaks.** While drinking is important for keeping hydrated, it also will help labour to progress as Mum will need to keep going to the loo and make sure her bladder is empty – again making space for Baby to be able to descend.

■ **Find a flannel.** Some women may experience lower back discomfort during this stage and using a warm flannel can help alleviate this (thus incidentally earning you lots of brownie points!).

Your role

Keep attending to the needs of your partner and reassure her. Subtly keep an eye on her contractions and note to yourself how frequent they are, how long they are lasting and look for them settling into a pattern.

A useful guide here is the 4-1-1 technique:

The 4-1-1 technique

A really good indicator for labour, which I usually use as guidance, is the 4-1-1 technique, which refers to contractions being:

- 4 minutes apart
- lasting for 1 minute
- been doing this for 1 hour

At this point labour is likely to be established. If you live a long way from the hospital (e.g. more than 20 minutes) you may want to travel in slightly earlier than this.

Remember – instincts override *any* technique (such as this one), so just use this technique as a useful guide. If your (or your partner's) instincts are telling you that you need to be in hospital or things are moving along quickly, listen to her first and foremost.

If you think your partner is in active labour, it's a great time to run her a nice warm bath. This is not for cleanliness, but because having a bath at this point can be helpful for two reasons. Firstly, water is a highly effective form of natural pain relief (see page 102), so if she is feeling any discomfort from the contractions this will help to ease that. Secondly, by getting into a nice deep, hot bath one of two things is likely to happen. If she is still in pre labour, the contractions may slow down, or even stop, for a while. If she is in active labour, it is likely to encourage the contractions to strengthen and speed up. So, Dad, once Mum is in the bath, stay close by; she may need your help to get back out if contractions do increase in intensity.

Now is also a good time to use those massage techniques if you have learnt any, but bear in mind that over 50 per cent of women are not that keen on being touched while in labour, so check first and stop if you are asked to. You can gently stroke her arms and her back. This will help her produce endorphins, which are the body's natural pain relief, which may help to minimise or prevent any discomfort.

Again, keep making sure that she is drinking. Have those bendy straws from your labour kit (see page 116) to hand and offer her sips between contractions.

Going to hospital

A very common question I get asked is 'When should we go to the hospital?' Dad, I know you can feel the burden of this one, because you don't want to go too early. If you attend hospital too early, the labour is likely to stall when you arrive (due to that adrenalin) and you are likely to end up going home again, with a possibly stalled labour. Think back to when I discussed the role of protector and how the best place to spend most of your labour is at home (see pages 72 and 120). However, more of you have a slight fear about the prospect of having to be midwife to your newborn due to not getting to the hospital in time, so I understand why you don't want to leave it too late either (more on that later!).

Timing the contractions can give you an idea of what is happening. You can use an ordinary stopwatch or, if you own a smartphone, download an app to help you keep tabs. Whatever you choose, don't get carried away with exploring all the features of the latest app or spend the whole time staring at your watch. Your attention needs to be on *her*. It's also important to remember that labours vary and if your app tells you one thing, but instincts tell you something else, ditch your phone and listen to those instincts.

You will want to call the hospital and let them know you think it is time – in all likelihood they will ask to speak to your partner – not because you are not a great conversationalist, but because by talking to Mum it gives them an opportunity to assess for themselves how far along she is.

My main word of caution when it comes to all this 'guidance' is not to let any of it override your instincts. *If your, or her, instincts say that she should be at the hospital, then listen to them.*

On that journey to the hospital you are likely to be feeling exhilarated and anxious. It can be pretty distracting to be driving a woman in labour, but stay focused as it's important that you all arrive safely.

Once you get there, park as quickly as possible; your priority is to keep Mum calm. If you have difficulty parking and need to dump the car or you don't have enough change, then make sure you leave it somewhere out of the way, and get Mum into the hospital without causing her any anxiety. Remember your role as protector and advocate (see pages 72 and 80). You should keep Mum as calm and relaxed as possible. You can always sort out a parking ticket later, and it's better to get one than miss the birth of your baby!

Transition

You will remember in chapter 6 on labour basics I discussed how some women can experience a 'transition' stage (page 66), where they may get physical symptoms (shakes and vomiting) or more emotional symptoms (self-doubt and wishing to stop).

The reality is that Baby should be here very soon and, as its name suggests, transition is temporary; the symptoms will pass. Now, if your partner does start going through this it can be very unsettling for her, so it is at this point that you really have to swing into action, and you need to be at your supportive and reassuring best:

- **You will get to use your full vocabulary.** You will tell her how proud of her you are, how much you love her, how it won't be long until you meet your baby and other positive, reassuring things. Have a think through in advance about what things you will be able to say to her so that you aren't sitting there repeating 'You are doing really well' over and over for 10 minutes!
- **Guide her through calm, slow breaths.**
- **Just be there,** hold her hand or place your hand on her shoulder, so that she knows she is not alone.
- **Keep the fix-it reflex under control** and do not start asking the midwife on her behalf for pain relief, because ... before

you know it, the midwife will let you know that it is time to meet your baby which means you are at ...

The second stage: the birth

This is the point that you have probably been most focused on. Mum is now birthing your baby and shortly you will get to see your baby in the flesh for the first time! To be fair, Mum is doing the vast majority of the hard work at this point, but there are still several important roles for you, which can make a big difference:

- **Support Mum in a good position.** The first thing that you will work together to achieve now is supporting Mum into a position that feels right for her to birth her baby. Hopefully you will already have discussed this and know which she would like to try, but check with her just in case she has changed her mind or feels comfortable in a different position.
- **Give encouragement.** Your main role during the second stage is to *calmly* provide lots of positive encouragement. You don't need to be shouting like a football coach or cheering 'Come on, you can do it!'
- **Definitely don't fall into the trap** of saying 'just one more push' as by the tenth time you have said this, she will want to kill you.
- **Have that flannel from your birth bag to hand,** already run under the cold tap, as she may get a lot of relief from having her brow mopped between contractions.
- **Have a glass of water** with that bendy straw to hand in case she needs a sip between contractions.

Then, congratulations! Your baby is here. Your role is not quite over with yet, though. Remember your birth preferences about what happens immediately after the birth (see page 108)? You need to just check they have been recognised and are being followed or, if they are not, understand why so that you can make sure your partner understands what is happening too.

Try to have a photo taken of those first moments together, so that you can capture your first minutes as a family together. Steph and I have a photo from the first minute after the birth of both our babies and it is an amazing memento to look back at many years later. Usually these photos will have Mum not necessarily looking her best, so they might be for your own personal albums rather than for posting on Facebook ... I'm not sure that Steph has yet forgiven me for when a post-birth photo of her was aired on primetime BBC! In fact it was this one:

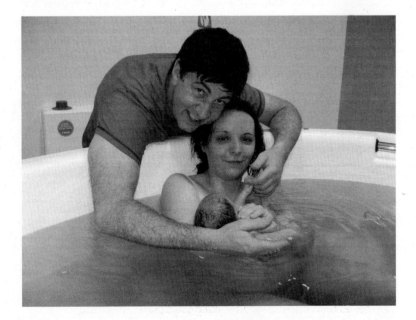

The third stage: birthing the placenta

Phew! You are nearly there. Yes, I said 'nearly'. In the heat of the moment it is easy to forget this, but remember – it's not over yet. Mum still needs to birth the placenta.

Hopefully in your birth preferences you discussed the third stage (because I told you to in an earlier chapter – see page 108!) and decided whether you wanted a natural or managed stage. Do choose a preference, but, again, it is fine for Mum to be able to change her mind on the day.

- **Make sure the midwives know** your preference for the third stage and check with Mum that she still wants to do this.
- **Don't be in a hurry to rush off,** even once the placenta is birthed. Enjoy these first moments as a family. Welcome your newborn, take time to hold her, tell your partner how proud of her you are. Let the world wait; those first few minutes and hours are so precious and you cannot get them back again.

'There were a few twinges that evening, but really nothing happened until the following evening on Wednesday. Joanne, my wife, had her first more painful contractions about 8pm on Wednesday. We were walking to the local shop, which was an excellent distraction for her as we were chatting to some neighbours that we met on the short walk. It wasn't until 10pm that Joanne showed signs of being far more uncomfortable. I then decided to time the contractions as you suggested. From then we went upstairs and I tried to keep her as comfortable as possible using some pillows, which she found very helpful. The contractions continued irregularly and became more regular about midnight.

Following what I had learnt, I did not telephone the hospital until 4-1-1, at 3am. They were helpful and spoke to Joanne and asked me to keep her at home as long as possible. We stayed at home for another hour and a half, when I could see that the contractions were becoming quite unbearable and that she might need some pain relief.

Keeping in mind the theme of serenity and calmness, I loaded the car at 4.30am with our pre-packed bags, some food and drinks and also the baby car seat. By this time the contractions were just over two minutes apart and were lasting about a minute.

I then drove very gently and calmly to Peterborough City Hospital.

After the short 15- to 20-minute journey we arrived and smoothly went through to the reception and checked in. Joanne was then monitored for a while prior to her examination. On examination the midwife was quite shocked and surprised to find that Joanne was fully dilated and ready to push.

We were then shown to a delivery room, which was very comfortable, and, after Joanne had had some gas and air, the midwife that had been assigned to us prompted her to push when ready. I was on hand to provide drinks and not ask questions.

After 15 minutes of pushing, her waters broke and we were told that there may have been some meconium in the amniotic fluid. Joanne then was aware that the baby needed to be out as soon as possible and a further five minutes of pushing was all that was necessary.

Our baby, Tamsin, was born at 6:31am on Thursday. I remembered the dos and don'ts of labour and *did not* rush off and make any telephone calls for a least an hour or so! Joanne had to be stitched up and this was quite distressing for her. I sat next to her and held her hand during that time.

I was extremely impressed at how effective what I had learnt had been, and have no doubt that without it our birth would not have gone so well.' — **Stuart**

case study

CHAPTER 11

What if things don't go to plan?

So you have your birth preferences, you have released and confronted your fears, you have your role and you are going to control your fix-it reflex. If your partner changes her mind, you have your code word – brilliant!

What could possibly go wrong? There are two main fears that dads have around the birth not going to plan that are almost at opposite ends of the scale. First up, that there will be a medical issue, the natural birth will go out the window and medical support will be needed. Second, that everything will go so swimmingly, that the baby will arrive at home and it will be up to Dad to do the catching! I will deal with both ends of these worries in this chapter, so read on ...

Medical assistance during birth

The figure quoted by the World Health Organization (WHO) and our own Royal College of Gynaecologists and Obstetricians is that 10 per cent of births require an emergency intervention. In reality, given that the Caesarean section rate alone is around 25 per cent, never mind when you add on all the assisted births that also take place, it is much higher than 10 per cent.

This would suggest there are many interventions taking place which are not 'emergency' – so clearly there is some scope for informed decision-making during labour and birth. Hang on, hang on, I hear you say. What's an intervention?

Interventions

An 'intervention' is literally anything that is outside of a normal labour and birth. So I am talking about inductions, vaginal examinations, pain relief, foetal monitoring, assisted delivery, third stage medical management and so forth.

The cascade of intervention

The reason that it is important to be informed about interventions is because it is common for them to have a snowball effect – this is called the 'cascade of intervention'. Simply put, when considering any intervention, one of the risks you must weigh up is that by accepting one intervention, the likelihood of needing further interventions, to manage the unintended outcomes of the first intervention, increases.

Opposite is an example of a possible cascade. It is possible that there would not be any undesired side effects, but it is also possible that the side effects could have been even more severe, with foetal distress and an emergency Caesarean becoming necessary.

Now let's be clear, I am not saying that all interventions are bad: far from it. Interventions absolutely have their place, for the births that do need some assistance. Obviously our access to medical support leads to lives being saved.

However, when interventions are being offered in non-emergency cases, the idea of this cascade of intervention is a crucial consideration.

One of the saddest phrases I hear a parent make about their birth is 'We had no choice'. Remember: you always have a choice about accepting any form of intervention. Sometimes

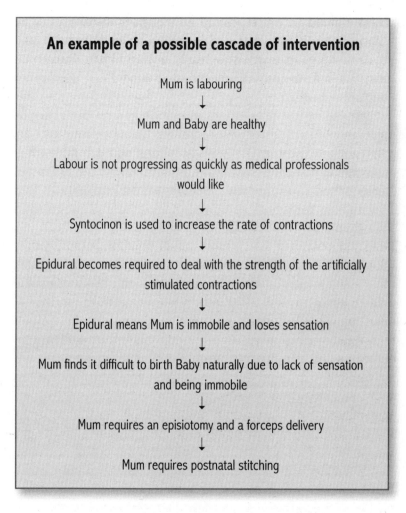

An example of a possible cascade of intervention

Mum is labouring
↓
Mum and Baby are healthy
↓
Labour is not progressing as quickly as medical professionals would like
↓
Syntocinon is used to increase the rate of contractions
↓
Epidural becomes required to deal with the strength of the artificially stimulated contractions
↓
Epidural means Mum is immobile and loses sensation
↓
Mum finds it difficult to birth Baby naturally due to lack of sensation and being immobile
↓
Mum requires an episiotomy and a forceps delivery
↓
Mum requires postnatal stitching

such choices are obvious as they are clearly necessary to save a life; however, in many cases they are judgement calls.

How do you decide whether to consent to an intervention?
So given that everything that happens is a choice, how do you make those choices? The system I am about to lay out is a simple tool, which if followed will allow you to make sure anything

being offered to you is part of an informed decision-making process. This is a great tool to use when working through your birth preferences, but it also comes in very handy should you be offered a choice that you haven't considered during the birth of your child.

Simply, all you have to remember when a course of action is suggested, or you are offered a choice, is to use your 'BRAIN'. First up, ask the medical professionals if you can take a few minutes to talk the suggested intervention through. If the answer is 'yes', then proceed through BRAIN (see below). This means that for whatever is being suggested you are going to ask for the:

B = Benefits
R = Risks
A = Alternatives
I = Instincts
N = Nothing

Now, this system isn't new or revolutionary and, in fact, it is the procedure that any medical professional *should* guide anyone through to allow them to give informed consent about their care. So working through each of these points in a bit more detail ...

B – First up, ask what are the **BENEFITS** to the offered intervention? How will it help your partner, your child and you as a family?

R – Next up, what are the **RISKS**? You must consider all the risks; what are the risks to your partner, to your baby and also are there any risks associated with your family later on? Can going forward with one course of action now restrict your choices in other ways later on?

A – Now that you understand what the benefits and risks are, you need to consider what the **ALTERNATIVES** are that are open to you. Remember – there is never only one choice (see NOTHING below).

I – Never ignore your **INSTINCTS**. What are they telling you? In the field of social work, one of the key things taught is to take heed of your instincts. Instinct is often your subconscious letting you know something before your logical brain has had time to work it all out. Make sure you find out what Mum's instincts are. Is Mum's instinct telling her that she and Baby are okay? Or are they telling her that they need some help? What feels like the right course of action?

N – Finally, you always have the choice to do **NOTHING**. You can always ask the question, 'So what if we do nothing for the moment? Can we just have a little more time?'

What is amazing is that following BRAIN is something most of us actually do every day of our lives. We will follow the procedure automatically, both at work and home, as we assess whether to do something or not.

Formalising this way of weighing up our choices is very helpful when you are in an environment that is outside your comfort zone. This gives you concrete questions to ask, so that you can become more confident in your role of advocate.

As with any tool, practise this before the day you might need to use it. Use it when you are working out what your birth preferences are; looking through options such as pain relief is a great way of practising using BRAIN before the birth. Get confident with the technique before the day you may need to use it for real – in an environment you may not feel as comfortable with.

Unexpected home birth

To reassure you – you are far more likely to arrive at the hospital in loads of time than have an unexpected home birth, although it does happen, especially in my experience if Mum has been practising and learning birth relaxation and hypnosis techniques.

These would be my top tips, should the situation present itself:

- **If you believe** that your baby's arrival is imminent (especially if your partner thinks she is pushing), don't bundle her into the car – it's warmer and safer to give birth at home than at the side of the motorway, and it's certainly easier for a midwife or medical support to find you, if necessary.
- **Call 999.** Although having a baby is not a medical emergency, having some support with you is! Tell them clearly that you are at home with no medical support.
- **They will ask** you what is happening and talk you through what you need to do (if anything).
- **Let Mum take up any position** she feels comfortable in. All-fours (see page 68) can help the moment of birth to be a little gentler and slower (if she is uncertain about doing it).
- **Just reassure her.** Tell her to trust her body and to allow it to do whatever it is doing. Just keep her breathing and tell her that you are there with her.
- **If you see the baby's head emerging,** just get ready with a towel to catch Baby as the shoulders are birthed. Don't touch or tug the baby while he is emerging. If you can see a loop of cord around the baby's neck (very common, and not usually an issue) you can gently unloop it, but *don't* pull on the cord.
- **When you have caught your baby,** pass him to Mum so she can put him on her chest. This keeps Baby warm, but also helps support his vital systems.

- **If Mum starts birthing the placenta** and you are still without medical support, just reassure her and let her body do the work. Make sure the 999 operator knows what is happening so they can advise the professionals on their way to meet you.
- **Then just wait for someone** to come to congratulate you! Leave the cord until a medical professional arrives and they will check over Mum and Baby to make sure all is okay.

'When I arrived at my DaddyNatal class, I honestly didn't know what to expect. I knew from the website that everything would be geared towards men and that things would run at a pace that made things easy to remember, but I was still apprehensive about what would take place — would there be any cringe-worthy role-play and breathing exercises?!

From the moment I arrived to the moment I left, things seemed to pass so quickly. I took in a wealth of information and actually remembered all of it! Dean had been great, informative, relaxed and friendly. All the dads felt confident to take part in the course and were happy to ask any questions.

I remember getting home and explaining everything I had learnt to Vicki. Neither of us had been on any other antenatal courses, so everything I had learnt was invaluable. I couldn't wait to attend the next course.

And then the next day ... Vicki's waters broke! Vicki was 34 weeks pregnant and had just left work to start maternity leave!

Luckily I had learnt from my first class that waters breaking does not mean that labour has started and I was able to remain calm and reassure Vicki. We attended hospital and, to cut a long story short, Vicki ended up being admitted to hospital and remained there until the following Monday.

During her stay at the hospital we were given totally conflicting information and were left feeling absolutely confused and bewildered. One obstetrician wanted to induce labour and another said it was too early. We had no idea what to do. I tweeted about how confused we were and got a reply from Dean asking me to call him.

Poor Dean must have regretted that – I spoke to him at least once a day while Vicki was in hospital. For me, he was invaluable. I was able to ask him questions about what we were being told and talk through other options we might have. I could then discuss this with Vicki and reassure her about what was going on.

Vicki came home from hospital on Monday 15th with the agreement with the hospital that we would return every 48 hours to check that Vicki had not developed an infection.

As it turns out, Vicki went into labour at home spontaneously the next day, and our gorgeous daughter, Lauren, was born naturally and quickly on 16 November 2011. It was easily the happiest day of my life. I didn't feel too bad calling Dean to let him know I couldn't make the second part of the course that evening!

I'm still so glad that I attended the class and learnt the DaddyNatal techniques. Without this help I know that Lauren's birth could have been very different. Now I'm delighted to be part of the DaddyNatal team and also helping other dads find out about everything they can do to support their partners during labour and birth!' – **Neil**

case study

CHAPTER 12

Labour
dos and don'ts

Trust me, guys! You need this! Having listened to so many stories about men getting into trouble while their partner is in labour and having guys come back and tell me 'You were right, I did X and it didn't go down well!!' No s***!! That will be why I told you not to do it!

So what will make everyone's life easier during labour – and get you out of this alive? If all else fails, follow these tips as a very simple guide to labour and birth. These tips apply to all types of birth; just use your common sense and modify them slightly, depending on your circumstances.

So let's keep this simple:

■ **Do as you are told!** Really! She really *does* know how she wants to be massaged or rubbed. And, yes, if she tells you to shut up because you are annoying her, then *shut up*. No, she doesn't need you to keep talking to her to 'take her mind off it'. Trust me, you won't achieve that, and you're probably just preventing her from staying focused! N.B. This rule *overrides all my others*, because if she is telling you to do something and I have suggested differently, listen to *her*. I do not want to be cited in any divorce cases as the third party!

- **Get into the driving seat.** It is likely to be your responsibility to get her to the hospital – if that's where you are having your baby. That means no getting drunk at the pub while you are 'on call', keeping the car topped up with fuel, and making sure you know alternative routes in case of road closures.
- **Be a Boy Scout.** Be prepared! Yes, I know she probably insisted on packing the bags for the hospital, but, as I said before, that doesn't mean you don't need to know what's in there and where it is! Make sure you know where everything is ... and *no* 'man looking'. Telling her during the middle of a contraction that you can't find something, when it is right there in front of you, won't go down well either. See page 116 for advice on what to pack in your own bag.)
- **Gadgets.** I know us blokes like gadgets, but don't get too focused on that contraction monitor. *It's* not having your baby! And trust me; she does not need you telling her 'here comes a *big* one!' It's not helpful for her adrenalin levels and, trust me, she will know it's a big one without your help!
- **Be Coach Sven.** You are Sven and not Sir Alex; you are not to shout encouragement from the sidelines at the top of your voice. Yes, she *can* do it, but she doesn't need you shouting at her. Be like Sven – focused, calm and offering support as required.
- **Extend your vocabulary.** 'You're doing really well, Sweetheart' uttered the tenth time in as many minutes will start to really irritate her. You, of course, will be proud of her, she will be doing brilliantly, she will be amazing and awe-inspiring. It sounds silly, but it's a good idea to plan in advance some different things you can say to show your support. 'I love you' or 'We'll soon meet our baby' are just as helpful for showing support. Oh, and anything you do say, say it *softly!*
- **Step away from the phone ...** During labour your total focus is her and her needs. Your text messages, emails, Facebook,

Twitter or even the football results can wait. Do not be constantly checking your phone.

■ **If it ain't broke …** Do not give in to the male natural instinct of 'fixing' things (see the advice on this topic on page 78). You will undoubtedly, at times, believe that your partner is in need of help. This does not mean you override preferences you have discussed beforehand and start deciding things based on your feelings. You need to understand that sometimes she will scream at you and sometimes she will swear at you. This does not mean that she needs you to take control. You have a job here as her protector and advocate (see pages 72 and 80). Stick to your birth preferences, which you discussed together (see chapter 8), and if *she* requests something, then use the code word to be quite certain (see page 82). Don't offer 'solutions', such as pain relief, to her, as this can undermine her – she will wonder whether you think she isn't coping (followed by fear, followed by adrenalin …). Stick with whatever breathing or relaxation techniques you have been practising and support her. That is your role; you are not there to 'fix'.

■ **Be the swan.** So, things are progressing and you are feeling what? Tired? Back hurting? Nail marks in your hand from being gripped? What are you going to do? You've guessed it – absolutely *nothing*. You are the swan: underneath you may be feeling all kinds of things and be paddling madly, but on the surface you are calm and just gliding along. There is nothing more annoying to a woman in labour than her partner moaning about how tired he is, or the fact that he is in pain! Keep your energy levels up and if she sleeps, then you can sleep too. Outwardly, you should be the picture of calm and support, so that her faith in you stays strong as her protector – and her adrenalin levels stay low.

- **The business end …** Discuss in advance if you think you would like some pictures or a video of the moment your baby is born. Some women will not want pictures under any circumstances, and again, despite what you might feel, you have to respect this – you are talking about her body. Even if you have agreed in advance that you do want photos, she still has the prerogative to change her mind. Do also make sure that you are clear about whether she feels comfortable with you being down there at all. She may not want you looking at her bits as your baby is being born. She may want you by her side or supporting her body in a particular position during the birth – again this is her right to choose.

- **It's not over till it's over.** Do not rush off straight after the birth to announce it to the world – the grand announcement can wait. Stay with her, get her a glass of water, give her and your baby a cuddle, tell her how proud of her you are and make sure she is okay. Enjoy these first moments you have together as a new family. When she is clean and settled, then you can sod off and go and tell the world.

- **Get the right facts.** If you are telling the world about the birth, get the info straight. Date, time, weight and name are crucial info. If you don't want to be inundated with a thousand messages asking for this info, get it right the first time.

- **Presents are always appreciated.** Some call them 'push presents' – not a requirement, but if you have a little gift for Mum (and one for Baby) it's a lovely thing to do. You don't have to give it to her the minute she has given birth, but having something ready to give her when everything is settled is a lovely way to show how much you care and how you have been thinking ahead to celebrating this moment. If you already have a child or children – make sure they give a little gift too – a special 'big brother' or 'big sister' gift. It is important to remember how they feel and show that they are appreciated too – obviously not just through material items, but also through lots of cuddles and special one-on-one time with you.

If at any time you are in doubt about what to do, always refer back to the number one rule: *do as you are told!*

section three

Life after birth

CHAPTER 13

Being Dad

Once your baby has been born, you will find that your life has changed forever. Your baby might be tiny, but once that little person arrives, his impact on everything you know is huge – especially when it is your first baby. Yes, one thing is for sure, being a dad is a whole new beginning.

Your next major rite-of-passage challenge as a dad is to get your new family home safe and sound. In all likelihood, you will be on an emotional cocktail of euphoria and exhaustion, so you are likely to be taking things carefully. You will probably triple-check that the baby car seat is safely installed, that Baby is nice and secure, and I'm certain there is no drive you will ever make again that will take as long as that first drive with your new baby on board.

What you may be feeling

When a baby arrives, as one friend put it to me at the time, 'It's the end of the world as you knew it!' It's true: life as you knew it has changed forever, but what an amazing change has taken place! For many of us it is a total (cliché alert!) roller coaster of emotions. Forgive my use of that term, but I can think of nothing that describes it more accurately.

You will very likely feel all, or at least most, of these emotions in the first few hours, days and weeks:

- **Love** – an overwhelming love for your child and your partner.
- **Fear** – fear of holding your baby, scared you might hurt him.
- **Happiness** – you will have days where you beam from ear to ear; life feels great!
- **Scared** – scared of being a parent; scared you don't know what to do.
- **Awe** – total awe at this amazing new life; this new life you made.
- **Worry** – worry about each cry, worry that your child is okay, warm enough, too warm, hungry, not hungry, needs a nappy-change, is bored – the list is endless.
- **Security** – you now have your own little family unit; you may now feel that your life is complete.
- **Tiredness** – and after a few days, tiredness the like of which you have never experienced before.
- **Jealousy** – jealous that *your* baby is getting all of Mum's attention.
- **Resentfulness** – resentful that you have been pushed out and your role has been reduced to fetching and carrying.
- **Pride** – sheer pride at your baby, partner and yourself, this new life you have created and every little thing he does.
- **Loss** – a sense of loss as realisation sets in, that life has changed and your relationship has changed.

This is not complete and I could go on to list just about every emotion under the sun, because the likelihood is that at some point during the first days and weeks you will feel them. What is important is to understand that all these feelings are totally normal.

Finding your feet in the first days

It is all the massive changes and emotional swings that led the renowned Sheila Kitzinger in her book *The Year After Childbirth* to coin the term 'babymoon'. She suggests that it is easier for dads to deal with all the changes by taking some time after the birth to just be with his partner and baby.

Those first days after Baby arrives are a magical (and yes, tiring!) time. And time is what you need in order to enjoy and adjust – time spent together as a new family unit, time spent gazing in awe at your new baby, learning about each other, learning new skills, bonding, experiencing a whole raft of emotions …

It's also a time to look at your new baby and consider what kind of father you want to be. Feelings of jealousy can be common, although these are usually temporary. Sometimes those feelings of jealousy also relate to longer-held feelings. They can be feelings of resentment for seeing your baby cared for or loved in a way that you did not feel you had as a child. On the surface it seems as though we dads are jealous of the connection between our partner and our baby, but often if we delve down into what has provoked those feelings, we begin to appreciate that they are nothing to do with our partner or baby at all.

What this can show us is how important our parenting is. How parenting has long-term influence on how we grow and who we become. It is worth taking some time to think about how you were parented yourself and whether that reflects how you want to parent your child – *because you have a choice.* Consider what kind of dad you want to be – not what you think is expected of you – and pursue that idea. Remembering how you parent will impact on how your child grows up; and the likelihood that he too will one day be holding his newborn baby, your grandchild, and considering how he was parented by *you* and what he learned from that for his own parenting.

This does not mean you have to be the 'perfect' dad or a 'super dad'; it just means considering what you want your fatherhood legacy to be.

How do I create my fatherhood legacy?

Everything around you is changing, so working together and teamwork are all so important. Communication between you and your partner is key – keep talking about how you both feel; don't feel pressured into expecting life to 'get back to normal'; make sure that there are lots of opportunities for you both to be hands-on with Baby to help prevent feelings of resentment. Life has changed and sometimes it takes a little time to work out how to realign all the new pieces of the jigsaw puzzle.

Most of us – and I am assuming this includes you, as you are reading this book – want to take an active role in the lives of our children. The thing is, being an involved dad is not just about playing with our child and changing a few nappies. It is about the whole spectrum of parenting and that includes our relationship with our partner, coming to a common vision on our approach to parenting and supporting each other in this.

One of the starting points for this journey is actually discussing with your partner what you think your parenting style might be. It is amazing how this is influenced not only just by how you were parented, but also how those around you parent. To work together as a team, you need to approach parenting together, remembering always that consistency is important for your baby.

So let's head to the basics – keep on reading for the essential information for those first few days and weeks. Make sure you have had a quick read through before your baby arrives, and then keep the book to hand for reference as needed.

Parental pressures

For expectant parents reading this, just be aware of the changes ahead and don't place too much pressure on yourself or on each other. It takes time for all of us to adjust to our new roles. Don't worry about what your friends are doing or not doing. All that matters is you finding out what works for you. Our modern-day competitive parenting culture means that people tend to exaggerate how 'well' (whatever that means) they are doing anyway, so there's absolutely no point assessing yourself against fictional milestones.

It is also helpful to think about what is really important in those first few weeks as you adjust to becoming parents. You need to be realistic and ignore what you believe others to be doing or what you think they expect you to be doing. None of us truly knows what happens behind closed doors and I have yet to meet the perfect parents, even after working with thousands over the years. This is simply because the perfect parents do not exist. We are all going to make mistakes; we are all going to do our best and we will all learn as we go along. Every one of our children is different; they are all individuals, so what may work for some doesn't work for others. There is a lot of trial and error in parenting – as you will find out.

CHAPTER 14

Babycare basics

What can you expect from your newborn? Well, in the first few weeks 'not a lot' is the answer. She will poo, wee, feed and sleep – and, while all this is going on, be bonding with you. Some babies sleep for up to 20 hours a day when they are first born, but perhaps not at the times you want them to! This can sometimes make it hard, as you don't feel she is ever awake long enough for you to really get to know her. However, she is getting to know you and, of course, there are things you can do with her and enjoy.

A newborn baby will feed regularly, probably every two to four hours initially. Allow your baby to feed when she needs to, as her tummy is so tiny at first that it needs regular filling up. It is normal for Baby to lose a little weight after birth and this makes sense as she has lost that womb environment where all her needs were being met around the clock – with Mum and the placenta doing all the work to support her temperature and nutritional requirements. Because this is normal, your midwife/health visitor may not weigh your baby again until a week has gone by, so that you do not worry about it! Your baby will also cry, but this is completely normal and it doesn't mean that you are doing anything wrong! A baby's cry is her initial key way of communicating a need – be it for feeding, changing, because of tiredness, or because she just wants a cuddle.

Practical baby care skills

So your baby is here, but how do you learn those baby care essentials? How do you change her nappy? How do you bathe her? How warm should Baby's room be? What about sleeping? How do you make sure she sleeps safely? There are many things to think about once Baby is born. In addition to what you learn here, do also consider doing a hands-on workshop where you can actually test out different products and skills (for information on classes, see the resources section on page 221).

Changing your baby

Which nappy?

Dad, probably the first nappy you will ever change will be your own baby's. Before you even start to change a nappy, first you and Mum will have to decide what sort of nappies you will be using. Will you be using disposable or real cloth nappies?

- **Disposable nappies** are incredibly convenient and come in a range of sizes and makes, so you can find the one which best suits you and your baby. They are light, easy to carry and don't require you to be organised with your washing machine – you just throw them away when they are dirty. The downsides are that they are expensive and not very eco-friendly (unless you buy the specific eco-friendly ones). They obviously also contain chemicals to help 'lock away' Baby's urine, which some parents are not keen on exposing their babies to.
- **Cloth or 'real' nappies** have moved on a lot in recent years. If you're like I was, your first mental image when someone mentions cloth nappies will be big bulky things that you pin together and boil to wash clean. Cloth or real nappies are now much easier to use, often with poppers or Velcro pads

for easy fastening. They come in a wide range of styles and colours, and you can even buy styles that last right through from birth to potty training! The benefits are that in the long term you are likely to save money over using disposables (especially if you are going to have more than one baby) and they are much better for the environment. Have a look around, try some out – the initial cost may seem high (between £100 and £300 for a kit), but in long run it is estimated that you will save nearly £2,000 over the period of nappy-changing your baby.

The world of poo

Now those first few nappies can sometimes be of real concern for parents as you watch the colour of Baby's poos go from a treacle black to mustard yellows and pesto greens before settling into the all-familiar browns (too much information, I know, sorry!). The consistency of some of these early poos can be quite shocking as well, from starting off like the consistency of tar, then becoming extremely runny. If you are not there already, I promise that no matter what you think of it now, there will come a day when you will be sitting around discussing your child's poo with other parents as though it's the most normal thing in the world!

The nappy-change technique

So, you get that whiff of a dirty nappy and you know it's time to step up to nappy-changing duty ... Here are the basic steps to changing your baby the easy way.

1 **Be prepared.** In the early days you might find that your baby does not appreciate having her nappy changed and she may cry while you are doing it. This is normal and it does usually get less traumatic, but as the weeks go by kicking legs combined with pooey nappies can make for an interesting

combination, so you need to have your wits about you! But don't worry, you'll soon have it down to a fine art!

2 **Gather everything you need and keep it to hand.** You will need a new nappy (or two), cotton wool, a bowl of tepid water and possibly a change of clothes to hand in case of a mid-change accident or if they have become soiled. Make sure Baby is in a safe place for changing – on the floor (but make sure she is on a soft changing mat and that the floor level is not too draughty) or on a proper changing table (never leaving your baby alone on a raised surface – you may not think she is capable yet, but the day will come when she can roll over, and off, a raised surface).

3 **When doing the nappy changing** for the first few weeks, you may wish to avoid using baby wipes, which can prevent the skin's natural oils building up and make your baby more susceptible to nappy rash. Using cotton wool and warm water is one of the gentlest methods to start with.

4 **Take off the dirty nappy.** Unfasten the nappy tabs on the front and then have a peep inside to see what you are dealing with. Bear in mind that as Baby's genitals (particularly boys) are exposed to cold air this can trigger a wee – so try to keep their bits covered until you are ready to make your nappy substitution.

5 **Clean the bottom.** Slide the old nappy out from under the bottom, and dispose of it by folding it up and refastening the tabs before putting it in a lidded nappy bucket, sealed container or plastic bag. Make sure that you wipe Baby clean with your cotton wool and water or wipes, whether they have done a wee or a poo. Check inside the folds of the thighs to make sure you have cleaned up everything. If you have a little girl, *always* be sure to wipe from front to back, to avoid risks of spreading infection. With little boys, *never* be tempted to pull the foreskin back to clean it. It will retract on its own, but not for a good few years yet.

6 **New nappy.** Slide the back of the new nappy behind Baby's bottom and waist, and then pull over the front to fasten. Don't pull the nappy too tight across Baby's tummy when fastening. While Baby still has the umbilical cord stump, just make sure this is outside the nappy. Some disposable nappies have a little V-shape cut out to help with this; otherwise you can achieve the same result by just turning down the top of the nappy before fastening it. Then dress Baby again and give her lots of cuddles!

Bathing baby

Bath time has always been one of my favourite times with my children and I think for a lot of working dads it's one of those special pleasures – coming home and having our own little time and routine with our baby before bed. Babies who are not mobile, in general only need to be bathed two or three times a week, as they don't get that dirty – being in one place all day! And between all the face cleanings and bottom changes they have, they are usually pretty clean anyway. But if you and your baby enjoy the ritual as they get past those first few weeks, then there is no harm in bathing them every day. Always make sure Baby is happy and contented before bathing, so that she learns to associate bath time as being a positive time.

Topping-and-tailing

In the first few weeks, or until the umbilical cord has dropped off, you can just do what is called 'topping-and-tailing' your baby if you wish. This method allows the cord to dry out too. Topping-and-tailing is a way of washing your baby without using a bath. Basically you can use a special 'topping-and-tailing bowl', which has two containers for the water (to keep things hygienic). You then bathe your baby while she lies on a towel. Dip cotton wool, a flannel or a sponge into one of the water containers to clean the top half of your baby, and then with new cotton wool, flannel or a rinsed sponge, using the other container of water to wash her bottom half. You can then wrap her up in the towel to be dried off. You can get some very cheap and great topping-and-tailing bowls, or you can just use one bowl but follow the routine by getting fresh water for the bowl between cleaning Baby's top and bottom.

Using a bath

You can bath Baby in an ordinary bath or a special baby bath – whatever you prefer. Baby baths can be used inside the 'big' bath, either with a stand or without. When your baby is still tiny some parents prefer to pop her into the kitchen sink. You can also buy special bath supports for small babies that are designed to leave your hands free for manoeuvring. Whichever you use, you will obviously want to make sure that you don't put too much water in – just a little (about 13 cm/5 in) is plenty, and that the temperature is suitable for your baby – 37°C (98°F). Lower Baby's legs in first, and use your arm to support her back, head and neck as she reclines in the water. You can then use your other hand to wash her body. Save washing her face to the end, perhaps even do this when she is already all wrapped up in a towel, with a little cotton wool or flannel dipped into the water.

However you choose to wash your baby, remember these top tips:

Bathing step-by-step:

1 Make sure you have everything you need to hand before you start – there's nothing worse than finding you've forgotten a vital item while you are trying to safely manoeuvre a wet, slippery baby. And you've only got two hands!
2 Wash tummy area, legs and feet.
3 Wash around your baby's genitals.

4 Wash neck, torso, arms and hands. Check all those creases under the chin and the armpits.
5 Clean Baby's ears. To do this, just wipe round her ears. *Never* try to clean *inside* them (cotton wool buds are not advised, in case of damaging the ear).
6 Finish off by cleaning Baby's face. Eyes first, gently wiping from the nose side outwards. You might want to have your baby all wrapped up in a towel before you tackle this part.

Once Baby is washed, pop on a clean nappy and clothes and have lots of cuddles!

Bathing safety

Check the temperature of the water you are using for the bath – it should not be more than 37°C (98°F). You can either use a thermometer, if you have one, or use your elbow. Dip your elbow in and you should not really be able to notice any feeling of warmth (or it can just feel slightly warm). If the water feels noticeably warm on your elbow put a little cold water in and try again.

Never leave Baby in the bath ever, not even to turn your back to reach something, even if she is in a bath support and seems secure. A baby can drown in a couple of centimetres (1 in) of water very quickly, so it is never worth taking the risk. If you need to leave the room, scoop your baby into a towel and take her with you.

Winding baby

Babies take in air as well as milk when they feed, but because they are pretty immobile when they are newborns they need a little help getting that wind back out in the form of a satisfying burp! Winding is one of the tasks that Dad can get involved in to support Mum and have a little time with Baby too.

There are a few handy little positions for helping Baby bring up her wind:

Over the shoulder

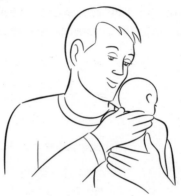

Lay Baby against your shoulder – you may want to use a muslin square to protect your clothing in case she brings up a little vomit with that burp! Use one hand to hold your baby in position and the other to rub up and down her back, or to pat gently. Keep your free hand on your baby's head for safety, just in case she accidentally jerks backwards.

Sitting on the knee

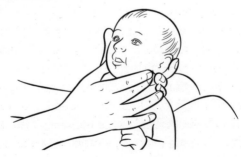

Sit Baby on your lap and gently rock her back and forth, making sure you support her head with your hands. You can do this by placing one hand on the back of her head (see picture) and using your thumb and forefinger of your other hand on either side of her chin to support the front of her head as you rock. Alternatively, sit her on your knee, leaning her slightly forwards, supporting the front of her head with your thumb and forefinger either side of her chin, while rubbing her back.

Tiger in the tree

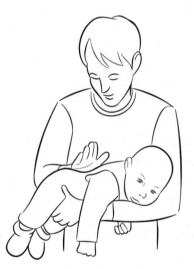

Lay your baby over your forearm, her head either in your hand (while she is very little – you'll know when she is too big, as she'll be too heavy to hold there!) or, easier, have her head in the crook of your arm, with her belly resting in the hand of your forearm. Keep that forearm close to your tummy, so Baby is lying over the arm but has the added security from your torso. Gently rub Baby's back. This move also doubles up as a fantastic baby-calming position – more about that later.

Sleep time

There are a number of things to consider as a parent when you think about your baby and sleep. Firstly, you need to consider where the baby is going to sleep, and how this can be done safely. There are various choices, and this is where you need to weigh up the options to decide what is right in your circumstances. So once again, you will need to engage your BRAIN (see page 134) and weigh up the benefits and risks surrounding these choices.

Safe sleeping

The recommendation from the Foundation for the Study of Infant Deaths (FSID) www.fsid.org.uk is that your baby should sleep in the same room as you for the first six months, in her own Moses basket or cot.

Whatever Baby sleeps in, she should have a brand-new, firm, flat mattress. If you do buy a second-hand cot, make sure you buy a new mattress, so that you are completely sure it is safe. The main things to be aware of are: it needs to be brand new and it must fit the cot. If you use a second-hand mattress it could have been in a smoker's home or it may be damaged in some way.

Do not use quilts or pillows for your baby until she is at least 12 months old as there is a risk of smothering. If you are using blankets, then make sure that they cannot cover your baby's head. Using a sleeping bag such as the Gro bag (www. gro.co.uk) for your baby to sleep in can make life a bit easier and safer – you can be reassured that she will remain warm enough overnight and there is no risk of her being smothered. General safe sleeping advice for all babies includes:

- **Your baby should always sleep on her back**, never on her side or front.
- **Remember 'foot to feet'** – place your baby with her feet at

the bottom of the Moses basket/cot, so she can't wiggle down and become smothered by bedding.

■ **Never put your baby to sleep in a hat** or with her head covered – this can lead to overheating. Babies also do not need a hot room to sleep in; the recommended temperature is 16–20°C (60–68°F).

■ **Do not put anything in the cot with your baby** – tempting though it is, and do not tie toys to the cot bars. She could become entangled or covered and items could pose a choking or smothering risk.

■ **Don't allow anyone to smoke around your baby** or in her environment – so it's best to ban smoking from your home altogether.

■ **Don't fall asleep with your baby on the sofa or armchair** – she could easily slip out of your grasp.

These guidelines are recommended by the Foundation for the Study of Infant Deaths (FSID) to reduce the incidence of Sudden Infant Death Syndrome (SIDS) also known as cot death. SIDS is rare and following these guidelines ensures that your baby is as safe as possible while she is sleeping.

Bed-sharing (sometimes referred to as 'co-sleeping')

Bed-sharing is exactly what it sounds like: bringing Baby into the parental bed. Now there is conflicting information surrounding this practice with regards to its safety and the risks to your baby, but many parents do it quite happily and there are some practical advantages, especially if Mum is breastfeeding. If Baby is sleeping with Mum, then night feeds become a lot easier for both Mum and Baby.

However, there are risks, so if, as parents, you choose to co-sleep with your baby you should follow these safety guidelines:

- **Baby should sleep on the outside of the bed** next to Mum – not between Mum and Dad. This is because Mum's awareness of Baby's presence is different to Dad's and the risk of Mum rolling on to Baby is far smaller. If your bed has one side against a wall, Mum should not sleep on this side with Baby between her and the wall because Baby could become crushed against it. Change sides of the bed so that Baby is on the outside unrestricted. To make co-sleeping as safe as possible, you can purchase co-sleeping cots, which fix on to the side of the bed, so you can keep your baby close, but she won't fall out of the bed.
- **Never place Baby next to anything that she could be squashed up against** or that could cover her face during the night.
- **Bed covers such as sheets, blankets and quilts should never be pulled right up;** you need to keep them low enough to ensure Baby's face is never covered.
- **Never sleep with Baby if either of you have been drinking alcohol,** have taken drugs, whether recreational or on prescription, if either of you is a smoker or if either of you is unwell, such as with flu or a cold.
- **Consider your baby's temperature when bed-sharing.** She will share your body heat as well, so do not put too many baby clothes on her or use a sleeping bag.
- **It is safer for mums who are breastfeeding to bed-share** with their babies than those that have chosen to formula feed. It is not recommended for formula-fed babies to bed-share with their parents. The reasoning behind this is that a breastfeeding Mum's awareness and sleep pattern is different. She sleeps more lightly and is more conscious of her baby's presence.
- **Do not bed-share if you are excessively tired.** This is because excessive tiredness can change the usual lighter sleep cycle mums are in.

- **Never sleep with your baby in an armchair or on a sofa**. Again this increases risks of Baby becoming trapped or crushed if you are asleep.

A lot of parents don't sleep with their babies all night, but take them into their beds for short periods. You must still follow the guidelines for both forms of sleeping if you do this.

Play time and bonding

There is a link between the amount of time a parent spends with their baby and how bonded they are with them – the longer you spend together, the closer you will end up being. Seems obvious doesn't it? However, it is amazing how sometimes us dads can forget this, and when we feel a bit pushed out, we go off and do our own thing rather than throwing ourselves into things a bit more. If Mum is the main caregiver, it might feel at times that she has a stronger bond with your baby, but this does not diminish the potential of the bond you can have with her. If you feel that you want a stronger bond with her, the first thing to do is to spend more time with her – getting involved in the day-to-day care of your baby is one way, but, given that most of us are really just big kids at heart, one of most dads' favourite ways to bond is through playtime.

Okay, so your newborn is not exactly ready for a game of football with you just yet ... but babies are sociable creatures and they will love having time to bond and play with you.

At first this play will be very simple. Try sticking your tongue out at your baby: you may be amazed to find that she mimics you! You can read to your baby, sing her songs or nursery rhymes, take a walk with her and tell her about the things you see or enjoy bath time together. At first you want to keep all these things gentle, and remember how quickly babies become tired. As your baby grows and gets older, play can become more animated, interactive and lots of fun.

Bonding is a continuous process – it's not one single moment in time. The first smile, the first time you make her laugh, the first time she says your name ... all these moments make you feel more connected with your baby and that bond deepens. Even with my children, who are now well past the baby stage, I still have moments when I feel that bond getting stronger. However you choose to do it, just take time to build that bond and connect to your child.

Routines?

I am not going to spend a long time on this, other than to say that there are lots of ways to parent and you have to work out what feels right for you and your baby. Some people swear by putting their babies on set routines for sleeping and feeding; other parents want to be more baby-led, where they follow the demands that their babies make. There are also some babies who fall easily into routines and others who do not. Every baby, parent and family is different, so you need to give yourself time to decide how you both feel on this one. The important thing is to discuss it with your partner and not let anyone make you feel guilty for not parenting their way. The last time I checked there was still not a 'right' and a 'wrong' way, or a perfect parent!

Again, it's not all or nothing with this one. You may find that you settle into a pattern rather than a strict routine, and as you get to know your baby, things find their own way. It can take time, but either way, do not feel pressured to conform to someone else's ideas and solutions – if it works for your family and your baby is happy, that is what matters.

CHAPTER 15

Breastfeeding

If, as a family, you have decided to breastfeed, you might think – that's it, Dad's job done … over to Mum! But this is not the case at all. If this is a decision you have made, then you need to work together. This is a team activity and your support is crucial. First up, let's bust a top myth: breastfeeding is natural and easy!

Yes, breastfeeding is completely natural, but for the majority of women it is not easy, especially in those first weeks. Establishment of breastfeeding is a learning process, getting Baby to latch on properly, demand-feeding and ensuring supply all take effort and can be physically and emotionally draining on your partner. Breastfeeding is about learning a new skill and it takes time, practice and dedication to make it a success.

There is one key person who can massively help or hinder this process … and you've guessed it, it's *Dad*! Yes, I said *you*. Strange as it may sound, dads are a crucial element to successful establishment and continuation of breastfeeding. Studies have shown that the more supportive their partners are, the longer women breastfeed and the more confident they feel about their ability to do so.

Unfortunately, some dads, without realising and without adequate support to take a positive role, can also be the reason for breastfeeding ceasing. So yet again, this is another key area where although it may be the woman who has to do it (much like birth), the impact of Dad's influence may have a massive bearing on the outcome. Time to feel that responsibility again, guys!

So why can Dads negatively impact on breastfeeding?

There are two main reasons. Firstly, it's that pesky male 'fix-it reflex' again (see page 78). If you skipped this chapter earlier on, I should really send you back to revisit it now, but, in essence, when us men see our loved ones in distress, pain or despair our natural instinct is to 'fix it'. And being men, we tend to look for practical ways to do this. Without proper support and understanding, this is what can make us men a liability! We don't do it out of malice, we don't do it for self-gain, we simply want to help our loved one and 'fix' the problem. In breastfeeding, this can manifest itself when our loved one may be struggling to establish breastfeeding, or generally just be finding it hard, especially in those first few weeks! For many men, if we see what we perceive to be our loved ones in difficulty, we will try to help, and often this will include (when all else seems to not be working) reaching for the formula. Why? Simply, because it is an almost immediate and practical solution – no other reason. We understand that breastfeeding offers the best start for our baby, but at the time our 'fix-it reflex' takes over and we want to help. The decision to formula-feed has been taken out of the hands of our partner, which can create a negative spiral of guilt, denial and then the very real difficulties associated with the impact mixed feeding can have on milk production … ultimately possibly leading to breast-feeding difficulties and ceasing entirely.

The second reason is a little more complicated. Now, us men, if not properly prepared, can feel excluded in a household of Baby and breastfeeding Mum. We can end up feeling like a bit of a spare part or a dogsbody. It's no surprise, really, if we don't understand what is going on or how us doing those little things actually makes such a massive difference in the bigger picture. If this continues, it can also turn to resentment, a feeling of exclusion and lead to male postnatal depression. Those early days, in general, are quite a stressful time, complete with the torture that is sleep deprivation for the whole family.

I'm sure many of us will agree, even if just privately, that at this time we didn't always act rationally, and again this is the case here. Generally it will be Dad that first brings formula into the house. Normally stating that it's 'just in case of emergency' or 'better to be prepared' or something along those lines. Men long for an opportunity to simply get involved with feeding, so if opportunity presents itself they will jump at the chance and often this is through the use of formula they initially bought 'just in case'.

Men do want to share that feeling; the one women get when they are feeding their baby and can gaze into their eyes, that moment of very special connection. We men can become very jealous of that connection. Once breastfeeding is well established, it becomes easier to actively get involved in feeding in a way that is not counterproductive to breastfeeding, by giving expressed breast milk. This would normally be possible a few weeks into breastfeeding, because if a bottle is introduced too early, your baby may start to refuse the breast in favour of a bottle. The other issue here is that breastfeeding is based on supply and demand, and in essence, the more Mum breastfeeds the more milk she produces. This means that if you are giving Baby some expressed milk in a bottle, Mum should still be expressing at the same time in order to keep her supply up – so the irony becomes that you feeding Baby has little benefit for Mum if she is still needing to express milk anyway!

So, yes, if you recognise those feelings of understanding the huge benefits of breastfeeding, but you are feeling slightly less enthusiastic about it now that Baby is here, you are not on your own. They key is to recognise this for what it is – that you feel left out or a bit jealous, and to tackle this head on. By following some of my tips and advice, you can ensure that you don't feel 'pushed out'. You will only be pushed out if you don't make the effort to support your partner and be involved.

Top ten breastfeeding tips for dads

1 Plenty of women feel very self-conscious while breastfeeding, especially in those early days. If your partner feels like this, then man up and get rid of unwanted guests in the house at feeding times. Also, if you are out and about, think about where you sit in cafes and public places. Make sure she can breastfeed discreetly if she is uncomfortable doing so in public – this is a great time to revisit your role as 'protector' that you learnt about earlier in the book (see page 72)! Mum can use a muslin or sling to give her privacy and provide a protective nook for Baby to focus on feeding and you can even buy special breastfeeding 'covers' that do the same job.

2 Your role of advocate is crucial (see page 80). Defend her feeding choices with family, friends, midwives, health visitors and anyone else who seems to have an opinion!

3 Go and get your baby for her, for those night-time feeds. It's a small thing to do, but she will really appreciate the effort. Once Baby has fed, you can take Baby again to wind and settle. This will benefit you both as often you will be able to settle Baby quicker than Mum, simply because Baby may still smell milk on Mum and make a fuss.

4 Help Mum by fetching and arranging her feeding cushion and supporting her to position your new baby correctly. You

can buy special feeding cushions that wrap around Mum to support her back and neck at the correct height and angle and support Baby in the correct position – otherwise you can improvise with ordinary pillows and cushions.

5 Get her a glass of water and place it in easy reach as breast-feeding is thirsty work and it's vital that Mum keeps up her fluid intake.

6 Bath- and bedtime are great bonding times for dads, so take charge of these routines. Make them *your* time with Baby as it will also give Mum a welcome break.

7 Try to carry your baby in a sling without your shirt on and enjoy some skin-to-skin contact. This will also give Mum a break – breastfeeding can be hard, tiring work.

8 Remember to compliment Mum on how well she is doing with the breastfeeding and how proud you are of her. Make sure she knows you are doing this together. Again deflect any negative comments and support your choices as a family.

9 When you have cooked her dinner (you are doing this, aren't you?!) cut it up into bite-sized pieces for Mum to manage while breastfeeding! It may seem strange, but babies seem to have the instinct to want to feed just when it's your mealtime too. Mum'll appreciate being able to feed herself easily with her one free hand.

10 If you have other children or people in the house, keep them entertained and busy so that Mum and Baby can feed in peace.

Above all, you both need to be involved to make breastfeeding work well. Try not to be jealous of that feeding bond Mum has – celebrate it! As in all things related to parenting, working together is important: your support is critical and will pay dividends for your whole family.

CHAPTER 16

Calming and soothing your baby

There is a school of thought that, for babies, the transition into our noisy, stark, colourful world can a bit too much for them to deal with. If you imagine for a moment that all your baby knew for her first nine months was the dark, warm, cosy, rocking, muffled environment of the uterus, you can begin to see what a culture shock our world might be.

Creating the 'fourth trimester'

By recreating the familiar conditions of the womb once your baby has arrived, you can help her feel more soothed, calmer and make her transition to the big world easier. You may hear this described as the 'fourth trimester', and it is simply about recognising that just because your newborn is now on the outside (so to speak) this doesn't mean she has forgotten all those things that kept her calm and soothed when she was in the uterus.

Sounds good, so how do you do that?

Skin-to-skin contact

In the uterus, your baby had continuous contact with Mum. Once baby is here, skin-to-skin contact literally relieves her of physical stress – it helps to stabilise her body temperature, heart rate and stress hormones, and stimulates the release of oxytocin – the love and bonding hormone – in you both. By supporting her basic physiological functions, you make her physical existence easier!

Skin-to-skin contact is exactly what it sounds like – get your little one undressed, take your top off and spend a bit of time having a cuddle. A lovely photo of Robbie Williams having some skin-to-skin time with his newborn baby was published in 2012, showing that this is something that dads can very much be involved in! You could also share a bath together – or even join a baby massage group to learn some lovely massage strokes to use during your skin-to-skin time.

Swaddling

Babies love the feeling of containment – and you dads love learning how to give them this sensation through swaddling! This is a favourite section in any class that I teach. Again, think about what your baby experiences in the uterus: that *constant* physical feeling of closeness and being contained. Swaddling is great for giving your baby that sensation of being held and contained, making them feel calm and secure, without you physically doing it. Having a cuddle has the same effect, of course, but sometimes you may want a break or may need to have two hands to do something else and swaddling is a great tool here.

Swaddling is something that was regularly used with babies from the day they were born 20 years ago or so and then the practice died out as there were fears expressed in respect of the safety for Baby and whether there was a link to cot death. Today, swaddling is once again becoming popular. It can be a brilliant tool to have in your toolkit as a parent, but, as with most things in life, you need to use your common sense and follow some basic safety guidance.

The benefits of swaddling have been studied. One notable study from Brussels looked at swaddled and unswaddled babies and found that those who were swaddled slept better. They also found that swaddled babies cried less, but when awake were more alert. You can either swaddle using a cotton cloth wrapped around your baby (check out www.daddynatal. co.uk for a video showing you how to do this) or buying a specifically designed swaddle blanket, which makes it all very easy and straightforward.

However you swaddle, there are some basic safety guidelines, which you should follow:

■ Never swaddle over Baby's face.
■ Make sure your baby does not overheat and only swaddle with cotton.
■ Always put your baby to sleep on her back, whether she is swaddled or not.
■ Do not swaddle tightly across your baby's chest.
■ Do not swaddle tightly around your baby's hips and legs; her legs should be free to 'froggy up' into a typical newborn position.
■ Don't swaddle a baby after three months of age if she has not been swaddled before.

As your baby gets older you may also want to swaddle her as a half-swaddle. This means swaddling her so her body and legs are still contained, but her arms are free. At about this stage, baby sleep bags also have a very similar benefit and are an easy transition to make for bedtimes. You need to be aware, though, that if you are going to use swaddles, one isn't enough. You will ideally need two or three. As with all things 'baby', one will be in the wash, one will be drying and the other one will be in use.

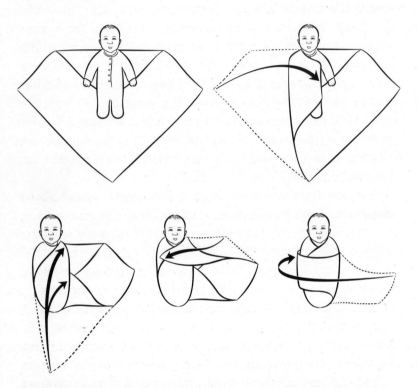

How to swaddle using a cotton square cloth. Half-swaddling is the same, but with Baby's arms left free.

Babywearing

Babywearing just means carrying your baby in a sling or a baby carrier. It is a great calming method, as it gives baby all the benefits of close contact, plus containment, and gives you your hands back! Be warned, though – you may become converted as you find out how easy it is to get out and about with a happy baby in a carrier and that lovely pram you spent a fortune on has just become an expensive shopping trolley!

Babywearing goes a bit further than this, as it also gives back your baby some of those sensations she had in the womb. If you think about it, during pregnancy your baby was used to a lot of movement. Think about all the times your partner was walking around, getting up and down, rolling over in bed, for example. Baby experienced all of this as a kind of constant rocking, and so movement is very familiar and soothing for her. Ever seen a baby crying in their parent's arms when they sit down, but the moment they stand and start rocking they quieted? Babies tend to love movement, so wearing your baby in a baby carrier or sling is fantastic for calming her down.

But where do you start? There are so many types of baby carriers on the market, including slings, wraps, stretchy wraps, Mei Tai's, soft structured carriers and structured carriers. The choices are almost endless and can in themselves be off-putting. The best way is to try a few on, go to a shop and get the staff to demonstrate them and try them out for yourselves. Do this before Baby arrives and practise putting it on at home. It is important that you get one you are comfortable with, otherwise you are not likely to use it when your baby arrives – it will sit in a cupboard gathering dust.

Dads, through babywearing you will find that your bond with your baby deepens and develops quicker. You also suddenly find that your hands are free and you can do other things while wearing Baby. I know plenty of parents who will put Baby in a carrier around the house, to comfort and calm her but to also allow them to get on with other things.

For a baby with reflux, babywearing can be extremely beneficial if you are using a carrier that keeps Baby upright, and using carriers also helps Baby develop those neck muscles used for head control.

As with anything, there is some basic safety advice:

- **If using a sling-style carrier for a baby less than six months old**, you should face her in to your chest rather than outwards. This is for a number of reasons, including preventing babies getting over-stimulated, but also to protect her face.
- **If you are wearing Baby in upright position on your front** then the top of Baby's head should be at about the same height as your sternum. An easy way to check is as follows: you should be able to bend your head forwards and gently kiss Baby on top of her head. If your baby is right in front of your face, she is too high; and if you are straining to get down to kiss the top of her head, your baby is too low.
- **If you are using a sling** as your chosen carrier, it is especially important that you check Baby's positioning. Make sure that her chin is not tucked down on to her chest. You need to make sure that her breathing is not inhibited.

Tiger-in-the-tree hold

This was covered briefly in chapter 14 when discussing winding, and it is a great technique to use to calm your baby as well. Revisit page 161 to see how it's done! I frequently use it with dads when teaching developmental massage classes as a quick and effective soother.

White noise

In the womb environment there was a lot of noise for your baby, but very different from what she hears once born. In the uterus she will have constantly had the music of white noise to listen to – the beating of Mum's heart, the whooshing of her circulatory system and amniotic fluid.

Again, you can replicate this for your baby – you can indulge that bloke-ish desire for gadgets and use this as an excuse to download a white noise app for your phone (any excuse for a new gadget or a fresh app!) or you can buy a white noise CD. The sound of a hoover or a washing machine also works just as well. Alternatively, that instinct you have to say shhhhhhh-hhhhhhhh when your baby is crying is also white noise and you can use that too. Just keep repeating sssshhhhh – but do make sure you are saying it more loudly than your baby is crying, so that she can hear you!

Finding what works for you

What works for one baby may not work for another – you need to get to know your baby and try out a few of these baby-soothing techniques to see what works best for her and what you feel comfortable using. You and your partner may choose to use different techniques, and as long as they work for you and are safe for Baby, that is, of course, fine!

Some of these techniques also work better when you combine them, since obviously every element you add makes this world more like that familiar uterine world. A technique I teach is to swaddle (or wear) Baby, then rocking her while saying shhhhhhhh. This can be a very impressive technique to demonstrate to Mum and an absolute blessing, especially when resettling your baby after the 2am feed!

CHAPTER 17

Getting to know this new person

Now you might have flicked to this chapter assuming that it is going to be about getting to know your newborn baby and that would be a fair assumption. However, it's not. This is about the changes that can happen to your *partner* – some of which can be so profound that at times you wonder where the person you knew has gone!

Changes in Mum

There is a famous quote 'Once a baby is born, so is a mother'. Now I know that many women feel they have become a mother during their pregnancy and that they make a whole host of changes for their pregnancy. But nevertheless, there is certainly something deeper that happens when that baby is physically here in their arms. Notwithstanding these instinctive maternal changes, Mum is also going through a host of changes as her body starts to readjust after the end of the pregnancy. The reality is that your partner may not be *acting* like her old self, simply because she is not *feeling* like her old self.

Emotional changes

Hormonal changes in Mum following the birth will have a great impact on her. Post-birth, she will experience a sudden drop in oestrogen and progesterone levels; her moods are likely to be unpredictable, ranging from elation and joy one minute to frustration and tears the next. It is these hormonal changes that also bring on the 'baby blues' (more about this later, in chapter 22). If the birth has not gone quite the way she thought it would, Mum may also be dealing with some disappointment or upset relating to this. Try not to get frustrated with her mood swings, as they are not under her control; just be there to support and help with the adjustment.

As dads we also need to be aware of Mum's feelings. It is common for women to be very self-critical and doubting of their performance as a Mum. In all likelihood, she may also start measuring herself against a fictitious ideal that is simply not achievable, perpetuated by the media. Part of your role as a dad is to support, encourage and reassure Mum that she is doing a great job. Trust me, she is.

Physical changes

Physically Mum is likely to be feeling a little drained, but in addition she may also be experiencing after-pains, blood loss, pain in her perineum and also difficulties going to the toilet.

After-pains

After-pains are simply contractions of the uterus for the first few hours and days after birth. These are actually a good sign as they signify that the uterus is contracting back to its pre-pregnancy size. Breastfeeding encourages these contractions (and many women report that they are then stronger in subsequent births), so it is worth bearing in mind that for those first few days, Mum might not just be working out how to breastfeed, but also be dealing with contractions at the same time! Sometimes these can be quite strong and Mum may want some pain relief or need to use breathing exercises to deal with them. Always seek advice from your midwife on what pain relief Mum can use, depending on your circumstances and whether Mum is breastfeeding.

Blood loss

Blood loss after birth is similar to a heavy period, but it can last for a few weeks. If Mum is not getting enough rest in the early days after the birth, her bleeding will get heavier and this can be dangerous, so she needs to make sure that she is pacing herself and not rushing around too much. Even if Mum has had a Caesarean section, she will still have this blood loss, as the bleeding comes from the place in the uterus where the placenta has detached.

Sore perineum

If Mum has had a vaginal delivery then there is a chance that she will have a sore perineum – more likely if she has had stitches. This soreness can be part of the reason for Mum's difficulties in going to the toilet. To try to ease the soreness there are a few things you can help her with:

- **Have some icepacks ready** for when Mum comes home from hospital. This can be extremely helpful especially in the first day or so. When applying them to the sore area, first wrap them in a clean flannel or tea towel.
- **Run a nice warm bath** for Mum a couple of times a day and let her just sit in it for 20 minutes or so. Lavender oil can also help with healing. To help it dissolve in the bath water (and not just float on the surface) add it to some milk first and then to the bath water.
- **If Mum can try** to start doing pelvic floor exercises as soon as possible, these will help with healing.

So what do you do to help?

It can be strange seeing someone you know and love go through these tricky changes. It is even stranger for Mum, who is going through them! Everything will settle down in time, some changes and uncertainties will pass, and the others you will work out along the way. What will ease this time for you all, especially in the very early days when things feel at their most delicate and vulnerable, is to just be there as a support for Mum and to take care of the little, though important, things.

My top tips for supporting in those first few weeks

- **Write it down.** Keep a notebook and write down the things that need to be done. List the household jobs you need to do, note the shopping you need to get. Simply by writing it down you won't have to remember it and you won't stress Mum out by forgetting. If you forget, it can be construed that you didn't think it was important – and you want to avoid that!
- **Use the internet wisely.** What can you change to ensure you have more time at home as a family? Do you do your grocery shopping online? If you don't, now would be a great time to start – many stores offer easy online shopping, often with next-day delivery.
- **Get prepared.** Get ready anything you can the night before, when Baby is sleeping; this will save you time the following morning. At this point you are going to have absolutely no idea how much sleep you are actually going to get, so if you can buy yourselves an extra 15 minutes in bed in the morning then it is worth it.
- **Do a job properly.** If you are going to help around the house, then *help*. See a job through to its conclusion. Putting all the clothes into the washing machine, washing them and then forgetting to get them out again so no one has anything to

wear, is not helping. If plates are dirty don't leave them on the side; wash them or put them in the dishwasher and *turn it on*. There is nothing more annoying for your partner than finding lots of jobs only half completed.

■ **The five-minute clean-up.** A quick pick-up of obvious mess to keep your home reasonably tidy is all that is needed. Also have a look at chapter 21, on visitors, for ideas on how to get them involved too.

■ **Ready meals.** It is really useful to have made up some fresh meals and have them in the freezer, ready to heat up when you need them, rather than having to cook from scratch in those early weeks. Stock the cupboards with things like soup, pasta and other quick and easy foods. Obviously try to make sure the meals are still nutritious and provide energy – you are going to need that!

■ **Don't suffer 'back-to-work amnesia'.** If you are returning to work after a period of time on paternity leave, it is too easy to fall into the trap of thinking 'life is back to normal' because you are now back into your familiar routine. You do need to be slightly mindful that Mum is probably now doing on her own what you had both being doing up until this point. On top of this, it's possible she might feel a bit isolated or lonely without adult company at home. We have all seen the cartoon of Dad coming home from work and the house in a mess and him saying 'What have you been doing all day?' I can hear you saying 'Yes, but that's not what I am like', but most of us put our foot in it and say something stupid at some point or other!

■ **Be hands-on.** Us dads, we quite often do things differently from Mum, but that doesn't mean we are doing it 'wrong', just that we are doing it differently.

So make sure you keep talking to Mum, because if we men feel criticised or unsure, we tend to withdraw. Often if I talk to a dad who is described as not really 'involved' it isn't because he doesn't want to be, but usually because he isn't confident to be. So ask Mum to show you how to do something if you are not sure. Explain to her that you want to do your fair share and are still learning. Both of you working together is the best for all of you, so if you want to do your best, talk!

CHAPTER 18

Newborn checks and support

It can feel a bit strange – when, at last, it is just you, your partner and the baby. It is very common for parents to say that they cannot believe they are allowed to take this little person home. It certainly is a momentous moment and you will probably have that epiphany-like experience of sitting down on the sofa at home, looking at each other and thinking 'what now?'

You are not completely on your own, though. You will be visited at home by the community midwife and health visitor, you can take your baby to the baby clinic, GP or back to the hospital if you have any worries or concerns. Your baby will be offered checks and tests to assess her wellbeing. There is support available as you find your feet – so don't be afraid to use it.

Support

Your community midwife will come and visit you all at home, usually the day after you are discharged from hospital. She is there to answer any questions you may have and she will check how Mum and Baby are doing. She will make arrangements to come back and visit you at least once again, maybe more. If you feel you need more visits and support, let her know – it's what she is there for.

Your health visitor will usually come and visit you around day 10. You may have met her already while pregnant, and she may be the person you meet at baby clinic when you go to have your baby weighed during the first year. Again, your health visitor is there to support you, so do ask her any questions.

If you don't feel that you can confide in your assigned midwife or health visitor, but you have something you want support with, then you can go and see someone else. The important thing is to get support if you need it, so that you can make the most of enjoying this time together.

Tests and checks

There are various tests and checks that will be offered for your baby. These will be offered in the minutes, days and weeks after birth. Any check or test that you are offered is a choice and will usually be medically recommended, but it is also important to know that you can refuse something on behalf of your baby if you choose to.

Here is the basic guide to these tests:

'Apgar score' (general wellbeing test)

Straight after your baby was born the midwives will have conducted the first checks on your baby, just by looking at her. They will have given your baby something called an Apgar score. This will be done within five minutes of the birth and most parents are not even aware that it is being done.

The Apgar score checks a number of different signs and allocates a number to assess your baby's general wellbeing. Most babies give no cause for concern, but if something is not quite right it allows the midwife to call someone else for further checks and treatment as required. The midwife will check Baby's skin colour, breathing, heart rate, muscle tone and reflex response.

Physical examinations

Your baby will have normally been offered two physical examinations. The first will often be done at the hospital by a paediatrician or a specially trained midwife. This should be conducted within 72 hours of the birth, so if it hasn't been done and you wish your baby to have it, ask your midwife. It is usually carried out again at about six weeks, when both Mum and Baby can have a wellbeing check with the GP. They will conduct a full physical examination from head to toe, but will be paying attention mainly to Baby's eyes, heart and hips. For little boys, they will also be checking their testes.

They will be trying to identify if there are any concerns in respect of problems with the eyes, such as cataracts or a rare form of cancer called retinoblastoma. In respect of the hips they are checking to see if there are any signs of hip dysplasia or dislocation. While listening to the heartbeat they will be checking for possibilities of congenital heart disease, and in boys they are checking to make sure the testes have descended. All of these are rare conditions, but if caught early then there are a lot of things that can be done, so don't panic about these tests; they are routine.

Hearing tests

Babies are offered hearing tests within the first couple of days of their arrival. This involves placing an earpiece in your baby's outer ear and sending clicking noises into the ear. The test is very short and the results are available straight away.

Now don't panic if the results are not clear on one or both ears – this is not at all unusual. Quite often it is difficult to get a reading from the baby – especially if she is crying. It doesn't mean that your baby has hearing problems, but it does mean that a second test will be offered.

The heel-prick test (Guthrie test)

The heel-prick, or Guthrie, is a test for various conditions and is done by the community midwife when she visits you at home. As the name suggests, the midwife performs a quick prick with a needle on the baby's heel, and then a couple of spots of your baby's blood is dabbed on to a card to be sent off for testing. The test is conducted on most newborn babies and will be offered to you when Baby is between five and ten days old. You can request that the test is done at a later date and it can be carried out up until the baby is one year old. You can also decide to only have your baby screened for certain conditions in the Guthrie test. It is not a case of 'all or nothing'.

Honestly, this is probably the test most parents hate and few can watch. But don't get the impression that it is unpleasant for your baby – it isn't. It is a little uncomfortable for her and the likelihood is that she will cry, but it is over very quickly. If you or Mum can feed or cuddle your baby while it is done, it is possible she may notice it less and be less upset by it.

The test can screen for five potential conditions, although not all areas of the UK always screen for all five. These are:

- **Cystic fibrosis.** This is an inherited condition that affects the digestive system and the lungs. Unfortunately it is still one of our most common inherited life-threatening diseases. That said, it is still a rare condition, affecting around 260 babies a year in the UK, which is 0.0003 per cent. There are somewhere in the region of 10,000 people with the condition in the UK, while around two million of us carry the gene that causes it. Fortunately with advances in medicine babies now diagnosed with the condition have a greater than 50 per cent chance of living past 40 years of age.
- **Congenital hypothyroidism.** This refers to the lack of the growth hormone thyroxine. If this hormone is not present,

your baby's normal growth won't take place. Early diagnosis allows early intervention.

- **Phenylketonuria.** This condition relates to amino acids in the body. Some babies lack the ability to regulate their amino acid levels. If this isn't spotted, a build-up of the amino acids can lead to severe mental disability as it can affect the brain. Therefore it is important to spot this at an early stage.
- **Sickle cell disease.** This, again, is an inherited condition that affects the shape of red blood cells and reduces their ability to carry oxygen around the body.
- **MCAD Deficiency** (medium-chain acyl-coenzyme A dehydrogenase deficiency). Another rare inherited disorder – this time the body is incapable of breaking down the fat properly in the body. Modifications to diet can help to ease the symptoms.

Remember: most babies receive normal results from these tests, which means that they are not considered to have any of the conditions tested for. You will normally be advised of the results by the time your baby is around six weeks old. The results will be recorded in your baby's record book.

If your baby does test positive for one of the conditions, you will be contacted as soon as possible. It may be necessary to carry out further tests to confirm the results or you will be referred to a specialist to discuss the condition and talk about potential treatments available.

CHAPTER 19

Paternity leave and work

What about paternity leave?

Paternity leave is always an interesting topic for discussion, and as I write this there is, again, talk of changes being made to entitlements. Paternity leave as it stands entitles dads to up to two weeks off after the birth of their child or in the unfortunate circumstances of losing a child after the 24th week of pregnancy. There is a government figure for the minimum amount of pay dads can receive. This statutory minimum is not great, but there are also companies that will still pay employees their full salary for those two weeks.

What I would say is that wherever possible make sure you take the maximum amount of time off after the birth of your child that you can. When our first baby was born, I rushed back into work after a week, mostly because that is what I felt I *should* do. I felt unsure of my role at home and thought the most useful thing I could do was to keep the money coming in.

What I learnt is that paternity leave is far from being 'wasted' time; you are giving yourself, your partner and your baby a valuable gift. Whether you take time off as paternity leave or annual leave – just make sure that you take some time in those early days to be with your new family. The first few weeks after your baby is born are such an important time for all of you as a family and the more time you can spend together adjusting and bonding the better, and the benefits will be there for a long while after.

Experiences of returning to work

So much has changed over the last few decades in respect of parenting and the expectations placed upon dads. Don't get me wrong; I don't mean just expectations placed upon us by society or our partners and families. I mean the expectations we now place upon ourselves as well.

Lots of these changes are positive and, in many ways, we are very fortunate to be becoming dads in the 21st century. We now easily have the option to be fully involved in the pregnancy, birth and upbringing of our child. This change is also being recognised in our own perceptions of success, as highlighted in some recent studies, that as men we no longer judge ourselves or other men simply on our careers and financial successes. Now, just as important is the role we play as dads, how involved we are and our work–life balance.

This in mind, the end of paternity leave can be a signal for the onset of another emotional roller coaster for us dads, as reality strikes and suddenly it's time for one of you to go back to work.

This can be such a turbulent and unsettling time for both of you. I think Alex (blogger, also known as Daddacool – check out his details in the resources section on page 224) sums it up in a piece he wrote for the *Guardian*[4]: 'When the two weeks were over, and it was time to go back to work, I felt genuinely devastated. I was torn between my role as the primary wage-earner in our family and my role as a new dad.'

But of course that is only half the picture. What about Mum, when she is left at home, suddenly alone with their newborn baby? Again, I think this sums up how a lot of mums feel: 'In the first two weeks of our son's life my husband and I were united in our ineptitude; together we got to know him and learned how to care for him. At the end of a fortnight he had to return to work, which upset both of us – he felt pushed out of the family circle and I felt abandoned. After five months of maternity leave on my own I found the structure of our parental leave had turned me into the experienced, expert parent and had positioned him as a less capable onlooker.' I think as parents we are often not prepared for these feelings.

Changes after the birth will affect both Mum and Dad on physical, emotional and hormonal levels. For Dad, the major change he will experience is a drop in testosterone levels of up to 30 per cent. This drop seems to be Nature's way of ensuring that Dad becomes a more stable parent. Interestingly even the most career-minded of dads suddenly finds that work just isn't that important any more – and you need to be ready for this feeling to pop up. This can sometimes lead to conflict in the workplace if Dad has previously been only too prepared to put in overtime and unsociable hours.

Mums can start to feel isolated and alone. Suddenly life goes from working together as a new family unit, a team, to suddenly being left to cope, increasingly with little other support. To me it is no surprise that nearly one in five mums suffer from depression during the first year.

For dads, suddenly having to leave their new family for large parts of the day can leave them feeling empty, guilty and sometimes resentful. For some men, the way they deal with these feelings is to pretend they are not there and that nothing has changed – expecting their relationship with their partner to go back to how it always was. Unrealistic – yes – but it is not conscious behaviour. Sometimes that resentment of Mum having this time with the baby, and Baby getting all of her focus, can make us dads feel resentment, even jealousy. Yes – it's true – we dads can get jealous of our own babies!

Sometimes we can actually start to feel left out if we are the one to return to work. Our baby is growing so quickly and instead of celebrating the little things they do when Mum tells us about them, we can start to resent the fact that we are not there.

How can you make the transition easier?

If you do go back to work, make time to call your other half during the day to see how she is doing, especially on the first day on her own. Show her that you care and you are thinking about them both. Find out what has been happening, so you still feel involved, even if you are not there. Tell her you will pick up a takeaway or will cook when you get home, and if you can, take her a little something home, even if it is just a bar of her favourite chocolate.

Plan to make the most of your days off – these are now your special family time. Ask your other half what she would like to do, if there is somewhere she would like to go, as new mums can suffer from 'cabin fever', especially if they are not yet confident about going out on their own, or are unable to drive themselves following a Caesarean section.

In addition to this, though, consider how you make things easier for yourself. Make sure you earmark some time for yourself at weekends to have some one-to-one time with your baby – whether it's you who gets up with him in the morning while Mum has a sleep in, or you go to a dad-and-baby group or a swimming class. When you come home in the evening from work, take charge of the bath and bed routine. It will give you that quality time with your little one that you have missed during the day (see also page 165).

Remember, Dads, that Mum may also find it difficult, or a bit scary, if it's Baby Number Two or Three, too, as being at home caring for more than one child is a whole new skill!

Daddy daycare

Of course, in some circumstances it will be Dad who stays at home as the main carer. While there are not as many men in this role as there are women, there is definitely an increasing number – figures from the Office for National Statistics released in early 2013 showed that dads now make up almost 10 per cent of those who stay at home to care for their children. As a stay-at-home dad, you may go through some of the same feelings as Mum may feel when Dad returns to work! However, there might be more specific challenges for you as a dad, such as integrating into mum-and-baby groups – usually you will get a big welcome, but you might still find it a bit nerve-wracking the first few times!

Of course, if it suits your family better for you to be the stay-at-home parent, then it is something to enjoy – getting to spend all that quality time with your child/children as they grow up is a great privilege!

CHAPTER 20

Sleep deprivation

So, it has to be talked about at some point: the favoured conversation piece of all parents (yes, other than poo!) is how much sleep you are, or usually aren't, getting.

'Okay, everyone tells you this, and you will almost certainly have received numerous "witty" remarks alluding to your impending lack of kip. But if you're anything like me, you have probably been quite blasé about it and have inadvertently ignored them.' – **Tom**

case study

Sleep deprivation is probably the most common response I get when I ask dads about what was the thing they had been least prepared for following the birth of their child. This is why Tom's words above not only make me laugh, but really hit the nail on the head. We talk at length about sleep deprivation in DaddyNatal classes; most people reference the warning, and I cannot believe that other classes don't also discuss it. I am just not sure us expectant parents get it. We all think back to our younger years and how we could party all weekend, surviving on a couple of hours' sleep a night, or when we have had to pull all-nighters to get a piece of work done. What we forget to also factor in, is this time around it is not just about being tired, but also about how emotionally drained we might feel, which compounds that tiredness anyway!

What is sleep deprivation like?

For those dads who want to have a sense of what being sleep-deprived with a baby might really be like – try setting your alarm to go off every two hours throughout the night. When it goes off, get up and do something for 15 to 30 minutes, then go back to bed and try to go back to sleep. Do that every day for just a week and see how you feel! Then remember that you have only been doing it for a week – and that's without all the added emotional elements as well.

Sleep deprivation probably puts more pressure on the family than anything else. We all know what we are like when we are tired – we are ratty, prone to making mistakes, are lacking in patience, we can be rude and can suffer from moodiness. So understanding that it is going to happen and finding some ways of alleviating the effects are crucial – for your own sanity and for that of your family!

Coping with sleep deprivation

So how do you deal with sleep deprivation? First up, don't be blasé. Going without sleep can be difficult, but once Baby is here, changing your sleep pattern and doing some of the following things, although they won't actually cure it, will certainly help deal with it.

Power naps

In one survey I did with some dads on this topic, I asked 'What do you wish you had been taught?' One of the answers I got was 'How to master the daytime power nap!' This is a great answer and more sensible than it sounds!

So what is a power nap? This means quite simply a nap, even of just 10 minutes, that can leave you feeling refreshed. A power nap should not be more than 30 minutes and this is probably where most of us go wrong; we are so tired that we effectively go right off to sleep. After 30 minutes you are likely to go into a deeper sleep phase, which can mean that you will have difficulty waking up and you will also find it harder to sleep at night.

For both Mum and Dad, learning to power nap is a great way to combat sleep deprivation. One of the oldest pieces of advice to new mums is to sleep when Baby sleeps – and it makes sense to do this rather than rushing around trying to get the chores done. If you are like my other half and you find sleeping during the daytime difficult, get yourself a blackout blind or an eye mask to use for your daytime power naps.

Reduce your caffeine intake

Another key way of dealing with sleep deprivation is to make sure you are not interfering with the quality of the night-time sleep you are getting. Most of us will reach for a coffee or caffeine support when we are feeling tired but need an energy boost during the day. However, if you are having caffeine after midday, it can still be in your system and actually make it difficult to fall asleep at night, making you feel even worse. Remember, a lot of things contain caffeine, for example: tea, cola-style soft drinks and chocolate.

Be patient

The truth is that there will be days where getting enough sleep is more difficult than others. It is especially tough if you have a very broken night's sleep and then you need to go into work for the day. However, as with so many of these things, it is temporary and it will pass.

Men! Try to keep that 'fix-it' reflex under control (see page 78) – the solution is not necessarily to 'fix' your baby and 'make' her sleep longer. Babies do wake up a lot when they are little, but as they grow they sleep for longer stretches. Patience and power-napping is the key!

CHAPTER 21

Visitors and social life

Meeting the new baby

Once you have had your baby, you are likely to find that all your friends and family want to descend and meet the new arrival. This is a tricky one. You will want to show your baby off, but you may also still want time in your own new family unit and an opportunity to rest and work out what you are doing. It is difficult to find a balance, especially if you have a lot of family and friends close by. This ultimately comes down to personal choice, but I do recommend keeping visitors to a minimum during the first few days, giving yourselves time to settle into being a family and just enjoying your baby on your own as a couple.

So what do you need to be considering when it comes to visitors? Firstly, for most of us dads, if we are lucky we may have some paternity leave after our baby is born. This time will fly by, so it is important to make the most of it, as this really is time you can never have again – so think carefully about who you want to share this precious time with. This is your time for bonding, and this time where you are getting to know each other is just as important, whether this is your first baby or your fifth.

Be the gate-keeper

Discuss together how you both want to handle visitors, who you will allow over to your home in those first couple of weeks, and for how long. Then, Dad, you can make those arrangements with family and friends – you are the gate-keeper and your roles as protector and advocate don't stop because your baby has been born, in fact they have just begun. These are your roles for life in respect of your family.

Use your code word

It can be hard just asking people to give you space and wait before they come and visit – there is such excitement when a new baby comes into the family. However, they should understand that your needs as a new family have to come first. If you do have visitors round and you want a tool to use in case it becomes a bit much for any of you at any point, you can use the code-word technique (see page 82) in a slightly different, but just as effective, way.

I have worked with families where Mum has had a special phrase she would direct at her partner, such as 'Could you get me a glass of grapefruit juice' and this was a signal that she was feeling a little overwhelmed and would like Dad to organise gentle encouragement of the visitors to leave! This is doubly helpful, as it gives you a way to communicate with each other that doesn't leave either of you feeling awkward or you having to interpret a 'look'. It also means that it will feel safer for Mum to have visitors around, knowing that if for some reason it becomes too much, she has a way of letting you know, without having to let everyone know or appearing to be rude.

Always back your partner up

In your role of protector, it is vital to back your partner up at all times. If you are having a disagreement over a parenting decision, it's usually better not to have this discussion with the mother-in-law sitting in the room with you. If people feel the need to let you know their thoughts on how you have chosen to birth, feed, care, carry your baby (and so on – you get the idea) as protector to your family thank them politely for their input, but say that after consideration you are doing this your own way and you are sure they can respect that. Then change the subject! Never make your partner feel as though she is outnumbered, even if someone says something you agree with. Always back your partner up.

If you are having visitors over, there are some top tips that might help you make the most of their visits:

- **Make sure that all visitors** arrange a date and a time for their visit – they also need to phone before setting off to see you, to make sure that it is still convenient for you.
- **If you do not want to be disturbed,** then take control. Put a note on the door saying you are all sleeping today and do not want to be disturbed. Unplug the phone if you have to. This is your time; make the most of it.
- **When someone says** 'If there is anything we can do...' – take them up on it! Get them to bring lunch or dinner, so you have one less meal to worry about. Maybe they could even help with the washing up after you have eaten. It sounds a bit cheeky, but if your visitors have had children themselves, or even if they haven't, they will understand and be only too happy to help!
- **Mum may still be uncomfortable** breastfeeding in front of people while she is getting to grips with it. If this is the case and Baby needs a feed, then you should make sure the visitors leave the room if need be, *not* Mum. It's her home and she should feel comfortable in it.
- **Everybody has an opinion** about how you should parent your child, including your visitors, and everyone will want

you to hear their advice. Dads! Keep your role of advocate in mind! Just thank them for any well-meaning advice, but politely explain that you have made your decision on what is in the best interests of your family.

■ **If any visitors come with a cold** or other noticeable illness, then it is perfectly acceptable to ask them to not handle the baby this time. Most people will understand that you are trying to minimise the likelihood of your newborn picking up germs, and that your primary focus is the health and wellbeing of your family.

■ **Don't pass your baby around.** Those early weeks are still an important time for bonding between you and your baby, and all the time your baby spends in your arms is increasing that bond with you. Therefore don't feel you have to pass your baby from person to person. If you want him in your arms then that's reason enough to keep him there, and there are plenty of benefits to this.

■ **Don't be tempted** to let people who have been drinking alcohol hold your baby – no matter how safe they say they are.

■ **Only let older children 'hold' the baby** if they are sitting down themselves and are firmly supported and supervised by a responsible adult.

Your changing social life

Having a baby can be a major adjustment for those who have very active social lives, as inevitably the social lives you once had have to change. In the first few months, just about every part of your social lives will change. If you frequently had people round to dinner or entertained at home, you may reconsider this – never mind all the work involved on top of looking after your newborn, there comes the consideration of whether your social activities will be waking up your baby!

Going out for a meal with your partner also brings different considerations. If Mum is breastfeeding she will not be able (nor probably want to) be away from the baby for a long period of time, so eating out is not as romantic as it might be, but perhaps it's more practical to choose somewhere baby-friendly and take your baby with you.

Something you also need to be prepared for is the simple fact that one of you may not be comfortable with the thought of leaving your baby in the care of someone else. Even if you have close friends or family to call on, you may find you do not want to leave your baby. This is totally normal and once again is just instinctive, based on the fact that through evolution we are pro-grammed to remain with, and protect, our young! Ultimately, if one partner feels this way it should be respected, as they are not going to enjoy the evening out anyway. If this is your first child, until your baby is born you won't fully appreciate your capacity to love someone. This may simply make the thought of leaving your baby with someone else inconceivable.

Dad, if you have returned to work, you will also find that every moment with your baby becomes so precious, especially as often your little one will be getting ready for bed by the time you arrive home. So given the choice of going out for a beer or having some quality time with your baby, staying home for bath time or cuddles wins out on most occasions. This doesn't mean you will have no social life, just that it will change as your priorities change. As your baby grows older, you in all likelihood will find your social life changes again, well, until the next one comes along anyway!

One last word of warning about your social life. Your social circle is highly likely to change, especially if you are the first in your group of friends to have a baby. It is a standard joke among parents that they no longer see their friends who do not have babies as much any more. This isn't really any surprise, since if you don't have children you can only be tolerant for so long when conversations revolve around poo, sick, feeding, sleeping and your baby's first smile.

In fact, if you have moved to a new area, or just don't know many people living near you (perhaps because you have always been out at work all day), having a baby can be one of the best ways of improving your social life and meeting people! There is usually a wide range of classes or groups open to new parents, so it is worth getting out there, since when you have a baby, you will naturally find you tend to associate with parents more anyway. If you try a group or class and don't enjoy it, or don't get on with the people, then look for another one. For dads, in an increasing number of areas now there are specific dad-and-baby sessions or activities being held at weekends, so that you don't have to miss out either. At DaddyNatal we run specific dad-and-baby classes, where the guys come and learn a little about baby massage while comparing dad notes on everything – so have a look at what is happening in your area and get involved.

No one is suggesting that you should ditch your old friends, but having a baby is a great opportunity to meet some new ones, especially as they will all be going through similar experiences and situations to yourself.

CHAPTER 22

Postnatal depression and the baby blues

Postnatal depression (PND)

Depression is a key topic and men often tell me they felt let down by not being told about it at other antenatal classes. Knowing how to spot postnatal depression in your partner, and what to do, is essential information, but not just that, it's also about recognising that new dads are at risk too. Yes, you read that right! Men can also suffer from postnatal depression. Officially in men it is now recognised but unfortunately still very little research is being devoted to it even though it is estimated that 3 per cent of dads suffer PND in the first year of their babies' lives. Personally I think that the figure is far higher – simply because dads either don't seek help or are not properly diagnosed.

It is really important that if you think either you or your partner may be suffering from postnatal depression you seek support. If it is you who are suffering, don't just assume that 'it will pass'; you owe it to each other to work out what is going on. In addition, it is common that when Dad has it, then so does Mum and women can be very good at masking the signs of depression. However, the good news is that there is support available to help you overcome it.

Having depression does not make either of you a lesser parent *in any way*, in the same way that catching a cold wouldn't – it is just an illness, not a weakness or a reflection on how much you love your baby. Really, looking out for depression is yet another example of where teamwork needs to kick in, and you should both be looking out for signs of depression in each other.

Signs of depression include:

- **Loss of appetite,** which may go with feeling hungry all the time, but being unable to eat.
- **Being very low,** making self-critical comments about being 'no good' at being a parent.
- **Feeling tired** and very lethargic, or even feeling quite 'numb' and emotionally detached. This kind of tiredness is not to be confused with sleep deprivation (see chapter 20) as it can be linked with difficulty sleeping, not getting to sleep and even waking early.
- **A general disinterest** in the world at large, no desire to do anything, or even see anyone, especially friends and family.
- **Unusual irritability,** which can link with feeling unable to cope or not bonding/loving Baby enough (this is a common sign in Dad as he can feel pushed out or isolated), which can lead to guilt and turn into a vicious circle.
- **Crying or feeling** like wanting to cry all the time.
- **Being hostile** or indifferent to their partner and/or the baby.
- **Suffering from** panic attacks, which can strike at any time, causing rapid heartbeat, sweaty palms and feelings of sickness or faintness.
- **Becoming very indecisive** and finding it difficult to concentrate or to make decisions.
- **Suffering from** physical symptoms such as stomach pains,

headaches or blurred vision.
- **Mum becoming obsessive** about the baby's health, or about herself and her partner. This can also lead to excluding Dad from caring for Baby.

If you are worried about depression in either yourself or your partner, the first thing to do is to be *there* for her. Ideally support her to talk about how she is feeling to her health visitor, midwife, GP or any other mental health professional she feels comfortable with.

The baby blues

Postnatal depression is quite different from the baby blues, which estimates suggest that around half of all mums experience. A mother going through the baby blues might feel very low and tearful during the first week or so after the birth. Again, this is one of those things that is caused by all the hormonal changes taking place in those first few days.

Mum may feel irritable for no obvious reason and get upset or cross. The blues can last for a few hours or a few days, but they are usually over by the end of the first two weeks or so.

There's normally no treatment necessary, but anyone going through the baby blues will probably feel better for some tender, loving care from the people around them – yes, that's you! Peace and quiet, with opportunities to sleep, are likely to help, too, so just try to keep the environment around your partner as calm and relaxed as possible.

What can you do?

Ask Mum what you can do to help, but understand that she may not have an answer. If she is crying and doesn't answer, it may simply be that she just wants to be left to cry for a while,

so allow her that space, or just hold her while she cries, resist-
ing the urge to say anything.

Remember that sometimes we dads can feel that it is our
fault or something we have done. Don't blame yourself if you
didn't do anything to cause it; it is just a natural part of the
post-partum period. However, *don't* tell her 'It's just the baby
blues'. It won't make her feel better. Don't try to diagnose or
fix it (keep that reflex in check, see page 78). Just remain your
supportive best. Buying her a nice cake to show you care
wouldn't go amiss either. Remember, though, that these signs
should pass in a few days. If they don't and you are still worried, get support from your health visitor or GP.

CHAPTER 23

Sex

Sex is such an important part of the male psyche, that, yes, it has two whole chapters in this book dedicated to it! All jokes aside, the reason I feel this needs covering is to dispel some of the myths and stereotypes surrounding sex – this time about sex after birth.

The sex stalemate

Men and women, on a subconscious level within a relationship, are motivated to have sex for fundamentally different reasons. Understanding this difference makes understanding sex after birth a great deal simpler. In relationships, the male psyche is such that we men look at sex and our sex lives as a sign that things are okay with our relationship with our partner. For women, generally the relationship has to feel good in order for them to want sex. From this you can see how the possibility for misunderstandings might crop up – Dad is feeling a bit pushed out and isolated because the new baby is taking up a lot of Mum's time, so psychologically he is driven to seek out sex for reassurance that everything is okay. If Mum is picking up on signals that Dad is not feeling okay in the relationship, then psychologically she is definitely not going to be in the mood for sex – stalemate.

Something that it is also useful to be aware of is that new mums can reach a point where they feel 'touched out'. When Mum has spent all day carrying, caring for, soothing and cuddling a newborn (which is exactly what newborns need), it can just mean that by the end of the day, she may be exhausted from that physical and emotional effort and has no energies left for her partner. This is not a reflection on you personally (hence this is why you need to confront and disregard that idea – that no sex means there is a problem between you), but just a reflection on the work and care she is undertaking and how she is emotionally and physically exhausted.

This fundamental difference can often be at centre of relationship issues and disagreements in these early weeks following the arrival of a new baby, which is why understanding what is going on is so important.

I often ask the men in my antenatal classes, 'When do you think you can resume sex after Baby is born?' Nine times out of ten, the reply will be 'six weeks'. A bit like the 'due date', this is an arbitrary figure that has been suggested by medical professionals, but which again leads us dads to having unrealistic expectations. It is the tendency of men to start counting down the days to resuming sex as soon as Baby is born. If you think about other issues covered in this book, such as how men view sex, how men can feel pushed out or jealous of their baby and even the possibility of male postnatal depression, having a date in your mind can bring further conflict, especially when you are tired and cranky anyway. The six-week figure is actually given in respect of when it is *physically* safe for your partner to resume sex, assuming that she has had a normal birth. This six-week figure gives no consideration to either your partner's or your own emotional feelings in respect of sex.

I mean, let's face it, us men are meant to think about sex from anything between every two to three minutes to 34 times a day, depending on which study you read. So if we are led to have false expectations about sex, given that it is on our mind so often, this is obviously going to cause problems somewhere down the line. In various surveys, one thing that comes across is that a lot of women resume a sexual relationship before they feel ready to. The reasons given are pressure from their partners or wanting to 'get it over with'. I'm sure this is not exactly what most of us want going through our partner's minds at the time.

Unfortunately, again, there are many publications, books, celebrities and even birth professionals reinforcing unhelpful stereotypes around the sex-deprived new dad. The picture painted is almost as if we are gagging for it and our partners are not interested. These types of stereotypes are not helpful to mums and dads, especially in the period after they have just given birth to their child. It leads to mums feeling under pressure and dads feeling as if this is how they *should* be acting.

The correct answer of course to the question I pose in class, is you can resume sex when you are *both* ready.

If you don't feel up to it

While I'm discussing stereotypes, contrary to general assumptions, not all men are 'gagging for it' in the weeks following birth. In fact, it is not unusual for it to be Dad who doesn't feel like resuming sex after the birth of their child, so if you feel like this, be reassured that you are not alone! This is especially the case for dads who have perhaps witnessed a traumatic incident during birth.

Subconsciously men can feel that it was their fault their partners ended up in that position and they avoid sex now to prevent it happening again. This is usually a phase that passes, but if it doesn't, seeking support from a counsellor to help manage those feelings can be helpful in moving past them.

However, this is not the only reason why dads may not feel like resuming sex. There are many others, including tiredness, seeing their partner as a mum now and not a sexual being, male postnatal depression and fear of causing our partner pain.

Waiting until you both feel ready is fine; but be sure to keep communicating, so that your other half understands how you feel.

Resuming sex

When you do feel ready to resume your sex lives, things are also not likely to just go back to how they were pre-baby or even pre-pregnancy. In terms of frequency, it is likely to be a little less frequent than it once was. According to a *Mother & Baby* magazine online survey, six out of ten new parents said they had sex one to four times a month, compared to five to ten, or more, times a month before they became parents.

In addition to this, there are a couple of more practical considerations, which you are going to want to know about:

- **Contraception.** Breastfeeding is not a guaranteed contraceptive. Trust me, I say this as someone with two children who are only 12 months apart in age! Frequent and regular breastfeeding as a form of contraception is known as the lactational amenorrhoea method (LAM). If properly done, LAM is said to be 98 per cent effective. However, this only works if a) your baby is younger than six months old, b) your partner's periods have not returned, and c) you are exclusively breastfeeding your baby on demand, night and day. You and your partner should have a chat with your GP after the birth to discuss contraception as there will be various factors you want to take into account, including which methods are safe if she is breastfeeding.
- **Oral sex.** Bear in mind that oral sex on Mum does carry a rare but important risk in the first couple of months after birth. If she hasn't healed completely (internally as well as

externally), there is a chance that you could cause an infection in her womb and vagina. There is also the possibility of passing air into any open blood vessels of the healing uterus, which can cause fatal air embolisms. This risk, also small, does exist, and is the same regardless of the kind of birth mum has had.

- **Discomfort.** If Mum has had any stitches in the vaginal area, even if it has been a while ago, she may still be sore, so take it slowly. Hormone changes can lead to vaginal dryness, so again for comfort, lubricant may make sex easier and more comfortable.
- **Body image.** Be aware that mums can feel insecure about their postnatal body, so just be sensitive.

Quick tip

I am reliably informed that moaning about not getting enough sex is under no circumstances a turn-on for women ... The truth is if she feels a bit more pampered and looked after, she is more likely to be in the mood ... although if you only do things with sex as an ulterior motive, this is also unlikely to work!

A recent Netmums survey[5] showed that just under a quarter of parents surveyed (24.3 per cent, to be precise) waited until between two and four months before resuming sex. There were also another 10 per cent who waited between five months and a year. Hopefully these statistics are reassuring, although they fly in the face of the advice I am about to give you, which is to stop comparing notes!

Every couple is different, every pregnancy is different, every family is different and every dad is different. Women don't all have the same experiences with breastfeeding. Dads don't all have the same experiences in bonding with their baby. Our babies won't all learn to smile or sit or clap on exactly the same day. And so, doesn't it kind of make sense that our sex lives aren't likely to correspond either?

Instead of focusing on what is normal or what everyone else is doing, it is much healthier to try to focus on what feels right for you both right now. Sex will feature in your relationship when you are *both* ready. So focus on being parents and let everything else fall into place when it is the right time!

Conclusion

That's it, the end. Or, in your case, the beginning of your journey as a dad.

I hope you have enjoyed reading this book. Keep it handy so that you can revisit and review the advice contained within it – not just next week when something new happens, but perhaps even for the next time you have that positive pregnancy test!

You need to now take positive steps to making the ideas in this book work for you. You need to do your research, discuss and write out your birth preferences. Don't forget to start the steps for bonding with your baby through the pregnancy, so that you all reap the benefits once your baby is born.

Reading this book should only be part of your journey. Read the blogs I have listed and see other dad experiences. Have a look at the suggested list of antenatal classes and resources (see page 221). Invest in becoming a parent. You will spend plenty on their nursery, nappies and clothes, but what the baby really needs is a calm and prepared set of parents. Investing in gaining that preparation is important and will be money well spent. Find classes you can do together, as well as separately. Try to avoid classes that subscribe to a certain method, unless it suits the way you are thinking about your journey.

Try to find classes that are about true empowerment of parents. You should be able to just receive the unbiased information available and make your own informed choices. This is what I trust you to do. I believe all parents, when armed with all the information, will make the decisions that are in the best interests of all members of their family. Nobody else understands the needs of your family the way you do, so nobody is better placed to make those decision than you.

Keep reading; keep researching. If you are going on forums, remember that other people love to share their own experiences, but you need to find what is right for you in your own circumstances. We are all different, so treat any advice with a pinch of salt! Some people write things simply looking for reaction.

Avoid competitive parenting. I see far too many instances today where parents are measuring their children against other people's, or comparing their births against those of others. One thing you will discover is that everyone has an opinion and believes that their way is *the* way to do it. Your pregnancy, birth and baby are exactly that: yours. Everyone is different, so there is absolutely no need to compare yourselves to anyone else. You child will sit up, roll over, crawl, walk and talk when they are ready and not before. He will do some things earlier than other babies and some later: he will gain weight faster or slower than others. So please, don't waste time worrying about it; just enjoy him. Time will pass all too quickly, so cherish the moments and don't forget to have a camera ready at all times to record the journey.

Finally I am always happy to help if I can, so if you have questions feel free to email dean@daddynatal.co.uk and I will come back to you as soon as I can.

Useful resources

Antenatal Education – websites and classes

www.daddynatal.co.uk
The website for dads. Here you can get in touch with me, read my blog and book yourself on to a DaddyNatal class!

www.babynatal.co.uk
I am also the founder (along with my wife, Steph) of the Baby-Natal programme. This is an excellent resource, which has lots of information on the early days with your little baby. We have teachers all around the UK who run Practical Baby Care classes for mums and dads, to help you both learn the skills to care for your baby, as well as postnatal workshops on topics such as Baby Sleep and Colic and Calming.

Other Resources

Action on Pre-Eclampsia
Information and support for those affected by pre-eclampsia.
http://action-on-pre-eclampsia.org.uk/

BirthChoiceUK
A website which enables you to compare the maternity statistics of hospitals.
www.birthchoiceuk.com

The Baby Show
Great shows held in London and Birmingham that allow you to explore the world of having a baby.
www.thebabyshow.co.uk; 0871 231 0844

Count the Kicks
A fantastic charity, doing really great work to keep babies safe. They provide information and resources to help you keep track of your baby's movement patterns.
www.countthekicks.org.uk

Doula UK
A directory of doulas in the UK.
www.doula.org.uk

The Ectopic Pregnancy Trust
Information and support for those affected by ectopic pregnancies.
www.ectopic.org.uk

The Foundation for the Study of Infant Deaths (FSID)
Information and safety guidelines on looking after your baby and protecting them from FSID.
www.fsid.org.uk

The Miscarriage Association
Information and support for those affected by miscarriage.
www.miscarriageassociation.org.uk

OnlyDads
Provides advice and support for single parents on financial issues, debt, legal issues, health, relationships and much more.
www.onlydads.org

The Pelvic Partnership
Advice and support for sufferers of Symphysis Pubis Dysfunction (SPD) or Pelvic Girdle Pain (PGP).
www.pelvicpartnership.org.uk

Pregnancy Sickness Support
Information and advice on sufferers of morning sickness and its extreme form: *Hyperemesis gravidarum*.
www.pregnancysicknesssupport.org.uk
024 7638 2020

British Association for Counselling & Psychotherapy
A register of qualified counsellors if you or your partner need someone to talk to.
www.bacp.co.uk

The Association for Post-Natal Illness
Provides support for mums with postnatal depression.
www.apni.org; 020 7386 0868

NHS
For NHS information on pregnancy, including diet, tests and checks, etc.
www.nhs.uk

Gingerbread
Information and support for single-parent families
www.gingerbread.org.uk; helpline: 0808 802 0925

Birth Rights
Provides legal information and advice on the law relating to women and birth.
www.birthrights.org.uk

Daddy Blogs that are worth a read

In the first chapter I describe how writing a blog is a good tool for bonding with your baby. For your own entertainment or inspiration, here is a selection of the blogs written by dads out there that I particularly enjoy.

http://alwaystimeforbiscuits.wordpress.com
This blog is written by Andy, starring his little boy, George. He says of himself: 'Although being a Dad is the one thing I am most proud of in my life, I did not intentionally set out to be a Dad blogger – mainly because I can never focus on one thing at a time! Despite this, I do talk about being a Dad most of the time because my baby bear has made such an impact on my life.'

http://first-time-daddy.blogspot.co.uk/
Written by Lewis, who I first met on Twitter, this blog carries the story of becoming a dad for the first time. It has now had to be amended slightly as Lewis is now dad to two children. He has a very self-deprecating style and you will enjoy his posts.

www.idads.co.uk
The iDad – Parenting: The Unconventional Way is a blog that light-heartedly describes author Jamie's life and experiences as a first-time Dad. He says, 'I have very little serious advice to offer, but I hope that by sharing my "not-at-all-exaggerated" experiences it will act as reassurance to other first-time Dads feeling their way into parenthood.'

www.daddacool.co.uk
Alex is dad to three children; two boys and a girl. He shares plenty of humorous stories, plenty of rants on parenting and a good few product reviews thrown in as well.

http://mutteringsofafool.com
This one, written by Ben, covers a lot of topics concerning his life. Like me, he has two children close together in age, so Ben shares that journey with us. Also as he describes himself as one of those 'crazy runner' types, he also documents how he shares fitting that in with being a dad.

www.itsadadslife.co.uk
David described his blog as 'a way of expressing what I was going through as my wife and I neared the end of coupledom and entered the world of parenthood! I wanted to see what happened when my life became that of a dad's. As well as putting my own thoughts down, I really wanted to create an honest record that other new parents may find helpful'.

http://diary-of-the-dad.blogspot.co.uk/
Tom, dad to two children, writes this award-winning blog about his own parenting journey. He was also the man behind the book called *Who Let the Dads Out?*, which features a collection of dad blogger writing.

http://reluctanthousedad.com
This blog is written by Keith, who also writes parenting pieces for many different publications and websites. Keith became a stay-at-home dad and shares that journey, but he also publishes some great recipes, which are worth trying out. His children are slightly past the baby stage, the youngest being six.

http://livingwithlc.blogspot.co.uk
Neil started his blog as an expectant father and his story featured on pages 137–38. His journey has taken him through DaddyNatal classes as a participant, through the birth of his child, to becoming one of our biggest supporters, and we are now very proud that he has become one of our teachers.

Endnotes

1. 'Ehrenthal et al., 'Labor induction and the risk of a Caesarean delivery among nulliparous women at term', *Obstet Gynecol* (2010)
2. Selo-Ojeme, D.O., Pisal, P., Lawal, O., et al. 'A randomised controlled trial of amniotomy and immediate oxytocin infusion versus amniotomy and delayed oxytocin infusion for induction of labour at term', *Arch Gynecol Obstet* (2009)
3. 'Amniotomy for shortening spontaneous labour', *Cochrane Review* (2011)
4. http://www.guardian.co.uk/commentisfree/2010/aug/04/ fathers-view-genuinely-devastated
5. http://www.netmums.com/woman/sex-and-relationships/ the-mama-sutra-let-s-talk-about-sex/ lets-talk-about-sex-after-kids-survey-results

References

This book is intended to be an easy-to-read guide for the average dad (whoever he is!), so I have intentionally not included lots of potentially off-putting footnotes and references throughout the text. However, I know some of you may be interested in reading more about the research that has influenced my work, and so I include this reference list for you. This is not an exhaustive list, and there is still much research into the role of the father yet to be done, but this will certainly give you a taste of the evidence base that contributes to my work.

On dads and child development
Clark, C., *Why Fathers Matter to their Children's Literacy* (National Literacy Trust, 2009)

Flouri, E., *Fathering and Child Outcomes* (John Wiley & Sons, 2005)

Magill-Evans, J. & Harrison, M.J., 'Parent-child interactions and development of toddlers born preterm', *Western Journal of Nursing Research*, 21, (1999) 292–307

Pleck, J.H., 'Paternal involvement: revised conceptualization and theoretical linkages with child outcomes' in M.E. Lamb (ed.), *The Role of the Father in Child Development* (5th ed.) (John Wiley & Sons, 2010)

Sarkadi, A., Kristiansson, R., Oberklaid, F. & Bremberg, S., 'Fathers' involvement and children's developmental outcomes: a systematic review of longitudinal studies', *Acta Paediatrica* 97(2) (2008), 153–158

Yogman, M.W., Kindlon, D. & Earls, F., 'Father-involvement and cognitive-behavioural outcomes of preterm infants', *Journal of the American Academy of Child and Adolescent Psychiatry*, 34 (1995) 58–66

On dads and newborn care
McHale, S.M. & Huston, T.L., 'Men and women as parents: sex role orientations, employment, and parental roles with infants', *Child Development*, 55, (1984) 1349–1361

Nickel, H. & Kocher, N., West Germany and the German speaking countries, in M.E. Lamb (ed.), *The Father's Role: Cross-Cultural Comparisons* (Lawrence Erlbaum, 1987)

Pederson, F., Zazlow, M.T., Cain, R.L. & Anderson, B.J., 'Caesarean birth: the importance of a family perspective', paper presented at the International Conference on Infant Studies (1980)

Scholz, K. & Samuels, A., 'Neonatal bathing and massage intervention with fathers, behavioural effects 12 weeks after birth of the first baby': The Sunraysia Australia Intervention Project, International Journal of Behavioral Development, 5(1), (1992) 67–81

'Influence of swaddling on sleep and arousal characteristics of healthy infants', Pediatric Sleep Unit, University Children's Hospital, Free University of Brussels, Brussels, Belgium, Pediatrics (2005)

On the importance of the birth partner
Diemer, G., 'Expectant fathers: Influence of perinatal education on coping, stress, and spousal relations', Research in Nursing and Health, 20, (1997) 281–293

Henneborn, W.J. & Cogan, R., 'The effect of husband participation in reported pain and the probability of medication during labor and birth', Journal of Psychosomatic Research, 19 (1975) 215–222

Johnson, M.P., 'The implications of unfulfilled expectations and perceived pressure to attend the birth on men's stress levels following birth attendance: a longitudinal study', Journal of Psychosomatic Obstetrics and Gynaecology, 23(3), (2002), 173–182

Klaus, M.H., Kennell, J.H. & Klaus, P.H., Mothering the Mother: How a Doula Can Help You Have a Shorter, Easier, and Healthier Birth (Da Capo Press, 1993)

Klein, R.P., Gist, N.E., Nicholson, J. & Standley, K., 'A study of father and nurse support during labour', *Birth and the Family Journal*, 8 (1981), 161–164

Odent, M., 'Is the father's participation at birth dangerous?', *Midwifery Today*, 51 (1999)

Tarkka, M.J, Paunonen, M. & Laippala, P., 'Importance of the midwife in the first-time mother's experience of childbirth', *Scandinavian Journal of Caring Science*, 14, (2000) 184–190

On dads and breastfeeding
Arora, S., McJunkin, C., Wehrer, J. & Kuhn, P., 'Major factors influencing breastfeeding rates: mother's perception of father's attitude and milk supply', *Pediatrics*, 106(5) (2000) Available at: www.pediatrics.org/cgi/content/full/106/5/e67. Last accessed 26 August 2006

Bromberg, B-YN. & Darby, L., 'Fathers and breastfeeding: a review of the literature', *Journal of Human Lactation*, (13) (1997), 45–50

Cohen, R., Lange, L. & Slusser, W., 'A description of a male-focused breastfeeding promotion corporate lactation program', *Journal of Human Lactation*, 18(1) (2002), 61–65

Freed, G.L., Fraley, J.K. & Schanler, R.J., 'Accuracy of expectant mothers' predictions of fathers' attitudes regarding breast-feeding', *Journal of Family Practice*, 37(2) (1993), 148–152

Jordan, P. L. & Wall, R., 'Supporting the father when an infant is breastfed', *Journal of Human Lactation*, 9(1), 31–4 and 9(4) (1993), 221

Piscane, A., Continisio, G. I., Aldinucci, M., D'Amora, S. & Continisio, P., 'A controlled trial of the father's role in breastfeeding promotion', *Pediatrics*, 116(4), (2005) 494–498

Pollock, C.A., Bustamante-Forest, R. & Giarratano, G., 'Men of diverse cultures: knowledge and attitudes about breastfeeding', *Journal of Obstetric, Gynaecologic and Neonatal Nursing*, 31(6), (2002) 673–679

Shaker, I., Scott, J.A. & Reid, M., 'Infant feeding attitudes of expectant parents: breastfeeding and formula feeding', *Journal of advanced Nursing*, 45(3) (2004), 260–268

Shepherd, C.K., Power, K.G. & Carter, H., 'Examining the correspondence of breast-feeding couples' infant feeding attitudes', *Journal of Advanced Nursing*, 31(3), (2000) 651–660

Swanson, V. & Power, K.G., 'Initiation and continuation of breastfeeding: theory of planned behaviour', *Journal of Advanced Nursing*, 50(3) (2005), 272–282

Wolfberg, A.J., Michels, K.B., Shields, W., O'Campo, P., Bronner, Y. & Bienstock, J., 'Dads as breastfeeding advocates: results from a randomised controlled trial of an educational intervention', *American Journal of Obstetrics and Gynecology*, 191(3), (2004), 708–712

On the changing role of the father

Dermott, E., 'The Effect of Fatherhood on Men's Employment', ESRC (2006)

Dommermuth, L. & Kitterød, R.H. 'Fathers' employment in a father-friendly welfare state: does fatherhood affect men's working hours?' *Community, Work & Family*, 12 (4) (2009), 417–436

Fisher, K., McCulloch, A. & Gershuny, J., 'British fathers and children' (working paper), (University of Essex: Institute for Social and Economic Research, 1999)

Peacey, V. & Hunt, J., 'Problematic contact after separation and divorce: a national survey of parents', London: One Parent Families/Gingerbread (2008)

Smeaton, D. & Marsh, A., 'Maternity and Paternity Rights and Benefits: Survey of Parents 2005', Employment Relations Research Series No. 50. (Department of Trade and Industry, 2006)

Smith, A.J., 'Pre-fatherhood, fatherhood and earnings: the price of parenting', (Paper presented at an ESRC Seminar), (University of Essex, 2006)

'Working Families Policy on Flexible Working', *Working Families* (2006), available at: www.workingfamilies.org.uk

Dads and paternity leave

La Valle, I., Clery, E. & Huerta, M.C., 'Maternity rights and mothers' employment decision', Department for Work and Pensions Research Report No 496. London: DWP (2008)

Tanaka, S. & Waldfogel, J., 'Effects of parental leave and working hours on fathers' involvement with their babies: Evidence from the UK Millennium Cohort Study', *Community, Work & Family*, 10 (4) (2007), 409–426

PND in men

Cowan, C.P., Cowan, P.A., Heming, G. & Miller, N., 'Becoming a family: marriage, parenting and child development'. In P.A. Cowan & E.M. Hetherington (eds.), *Family Transitions: Advances in Family Research* (Lawrence Erlbaum, 1991)

Madsen, S.A., 'Fathers and postnatal depression: research results from the Project: Men's Psychological Transition to Fatherhood – Mood Disorders in Men Becoming Fathers', Rigshospitalet (2006)

Paulson, J.F., Keefe, H.A. & Leiferman, J.A., 'Negative effects of maternal and paternal depression on early language' (paper presented at the 2007 Annual Conference of the American Psychological Association) (2007)

Schumacher, M., Zubaran, C. & White, G., 'Bringing birth-related paternal depression to the fore', *Women Birth*, 21(2), (2008)

Wee, K.Y., Skouteris, J., Pier, C., Richardson, B. & Milgrom, J., 'Correlates of ante- and postnatal depression in fathers: a systematic review', *Journal of Affective Discord* (2010)

PND in women

GMTV Survey (2009) 'Unhappy mums'. www.gm.tv/lifestyle/health/essentials/dr-hilarys-surgery/post-natal-depression/19829-unhappy-mums.html

Holopainen, D., 'The experience of seeking help for postnatal depression', *Australian Journal of Advanced Nursing*, 19(3), (2002), 39–44

Acknowledgements

This journey is still only beginning but it has been an interesting one. There has been some fantastic support from various people so I would like to acknowledge that support.

Firstly, to my beautiful wife, Steph, whose support, input, patience and belief have made anything I do possible; her own passion in supporting expectant and new parents continues to inspire me. Secondly, to Sue Atkins, who has always been supportive of our work and without whom this book might still be in the pipeline. Thirdly, to Louise Francis, my commissioning editor at Random House, whose belief in the book from day one and support and patience has helped turn my work into this book for expectant and new dads.

A huge thank you also goes to Penny Brett, Head of Midwifery at Peterborough City Hospital for her belief in supporting dads as part of supporting families and for her courage in taking the decision to provide DaddyNatal classes to the fortunate expectant dads in her area.

Also Nicole Muller gets a special mention for her belief in all the work we do with expectant parents and bringing our workshops to parents at The Baby Shows.

To everyone at Baby Bjorn for their support of our work since very early days, for their passion in including dads in everything they do and for always providing positive reinforcement of dads in their advertising.

To all our Natal Company teachers around the country for their passion, belief and dedication to providing non-judge-mental and unbiased support, allowing more parents to make truly informed choices.

I know I will have missed people that deserve a mention, and I'm sorry, but I would like to also say thank you and well done to all the birth professionals, midwives and support workers that have supported our work and also share in our vision of supporting families through supporting dads.

Index

About the author

Dean Beaumont is a father of two and a leading expert in working with expectant fathers. He is the founder of the unique, award-winning programme for men: DaddyNatal. The only programme run by professional male antenatal educators, it focuses on supplying men with the support and information to prepare them for their role in childbirth and as a father. Dean has a diploma in childbirth education and frequently speaks at events and contributes to features. He won 'Best Dadpreneur' in 2011 at the Mumpreneur UK awards and 'Business Parent of the Year' at the Mum and Working Awards.

www.daddynatal.co.uk